Contents

by James Edmond O'Brien

1 You Are What You Eat

Nature supplies everything necessary to keep us alive, fit and well. Plants supply the staff of life; if it grows in the ground, on stalks or in trees, it's likely to be good for us. Together with poultry, meat and fish, shoots, buds, flowers, seeds, nuts, fruits and roots, they nourish all of humankind.

The whole plan is laid out for us. We just have to obey nature — and in nature, the general rule is that simpler is better.

But some foods are more than mere nourishment that keep body and soul together. Some are remarkable foods that come entwined in history and mystery, along with medicinal value and quite astonishing healing power.

Garlic, more than any other gift of nature, tops that long list quite easily. Its folklore goes back thousands of years, and continues today to fascinate us with both its remarkable power to maintain and restore health, and its stunning impact on cuisines on every continent.

Vinegar, though without quite the same mystique and written history as garlic, possesses a similarly remarkable range of properties that have proven of enormous benefit. In cooking, as a powerful health aid, and as a household cleaner and deodorizer that is not environmentally harmful — an increasingly important plus today — vinegars win high marks.

Other natural wonders such as honey, seaweed, fruits like apples and strawberries, and a long list of herbs offer such powerful aids to health and healing that they should be as important a part of our regular diet as our daily bread. They are inexpensive, easy to find, and promise an infinitely preferable route to maintaining health than any trip to a doctor's office or pharmacy.

The folklore and history surrounding these foods make fascinating conversation pieces in themselves. But it is when we add them to our diet that they truly shine. For it is only then that we can really appreciate them and their stunning gifts of vital vitamins, minerals and trace elements that are essential to long life and vitality. These fabulous nutrients from Mother Nature's laboratory must leave the big chemical companies absolutely green with envy.

Nothing they can offer from their multimillion dollar laboratories and sprawling factories can compare. And in this age of apparent plenty when much of the food we eat is sadly lacking in optimum nutritional value, these wonders of nature are the best means for all of us to make sure that we give our bodies, and ourselves, the chance to make the absolute most of this wonderful gift of life.

The Basics of Good Health

The ancient sages and physicians well understood the powerful link between food and health. "You must follow nature, and when you eat what nature offers, the reward is long life, happiness, health, wealth and prosperity," a consultant who became a dear friend, used to say. This remarkable man was Dr. George Blodgett, a physician and nutritionist, scientist and naturalist of national repute, who surely knew what he was talking about. He lived to the ripe old age of 94, practicing what he preached about nutrition and health until he died, and savoring every moment of his long and vigorous life.

He, like many other healers committed to natural health through natural living, recommended these very simple rules for good health: Eat a clove of garlic a day; drink two teaspoons of apple cider vinegar in a glass of warm water every morning and every evening; and add a teaspoon of honey. For additional taste, he suggested, add a squeeze of lemon juice.

This was his prescription for good health because his lifelong research into health and nutrition had clearly demonstrated, he said, that these foods supply all of the biochemicals, the vitamins and minerals, in the right balance of acid and alkalinity, to sustain life and promote health.

For many years he, and those who supported his views, were regarded as somewhat eccentric, to say the least, by the great majority of the medical profession. It is ironic that it was only in the last few years of his life, clinical researchers were, grudgingly, beginning to accept that he had been right on target all along.

2 The Stinking Rose

With all of the impressive findings that scientists have made about garlic since the 1920s, it frankly should not come as any surprise at all if we discovered that it truly does repel vampires, just like all those vampire — and Dracula — stories report.

Few foods possess as richly glowing a past and as detailed a history. Garlic is as close as anything in the world of edibles to being the universal food — almost every culture in the world uses it in some way in its cuisine. Incredibly, it has inspired poems and songs; and it enjoys a truly impressive reputation as a powerful healing agent.

Scientists have already taken the folklore seriously enough to study it at length. And perhaps to no one's surprise more than their own, in a remarkable number of instances they have verified all of the claims handed down through the centuries in folk healers' literature and old wives' tales.

So there seems to be no question that these claims are true all right, proven in laboratory and clinical settings. But that, frankly, is simply not the half of it. Entire books have been written about this humble looking bulb by reputable authors. There is even a garlic appreciation society — called, of all things, *Lovers of the Stinking Rose* — organized to extoll its wonders.

Every year there are festivals held to praise it, where its worshippers swap stories about new uses, favorite recipes, and the most effective methods of farming it.

And its success in the marketplace underscores all of this pomp and circumstance. It is the second (after pepper) most popular spice in North America. Think about it for a moment.. it's in so many of the things we eat — chips, dips, powders, spreads, sauces, flakes, purees, and all kinds of concentrates.

That Breath Factor

And most of all, it tastes so absolutely wonderful. Unfortunately, as with most things worthwhile in life, there's a down-side too — it's not as simple as garlic tasting good, because it can also make us smell very, very bad.

Which brings us, immediately, to garlic breath. Of course, most of us could do without that, but the reality is that if everybody in the country ate garlic none of us would notice it very much. It would be so much a part of all of our lives that it would become, believe it or not, virtually unnoticeable!

That lingering, clinging, all-pervasive odor is created by essential oils in the garlic bulb. These oils enter your bloodstream and circulate for a quite a long time — up to several hours. This is, at one and the same time, the blessing and the curse of garlic, because it is these oils circulating in the bloodstream that make the garlic work its many therapeutic wonders on us. And while it does that, it produces the characteristic odor that simply refuses to go away no matter what we try. That is because the source of the smell is deep into our bloodstream. Mouthwash, toothbrushing or chewing gum are all destined for failure against the dreaded garlic breath.

You may mask the smell on your breath for a little while — just as long as that minty toothpaste keeps *its* smell — but that won't outlast the garlic for very long. After that, as you may have discovered through experience, that garlic odor will come right back, leaking out of the pores of your skin, and you're right back to square one.

I recall living in the south of France for several months, more than ten years ago. Garlic is perhaps even more widely usd in everyday cooking there than in Italy itself. Climbing aboard the packed public buses and trains after a long, lazy lunch on hot summer afternoons could make even a grown man swoon as the contented hoardes exhaled powerful garlic odors as they headed back to their workplaces. But, oddly perhaps, I did not find it offensive. Perhaps that was because I was never one to pass up a chance to eat any dish well-laden with garlic either. And so the breath of my travelling companions was almost certainly no different from my own.

But despite the bad breath rap it has here, garlic can actually perfume the air. During the process of cooking, the odor of garlic teases the senses with a magical, mouth-watering fragrance. Just try walking through any Italian restaurant kitchen and breathe in that garlic aroma that wafts from pots on the stove and casseroles in the oven. It truly is a glorious delight.

All of this, somewhat serious, discussion tends to overshadow the lighter side of the garlic story. For centuries in Asia and ancient Rome, it has enjoyed a reputation as an aphrodisiac. So far we have been unable to locate any serious, scientific study that supports that reputation, but it is worth bearing in mind that old wives' tales frequently have more than a grain of truth to them!

The Plant Itself

Garlic is described in horticultural manuals as a culinary herb. It's a member of the lily family and it is very easy to grow at home. The technical Latin name is *allium sativum*, which categorizes garlic as a hardy perennial bulb. It is a first cousin to the family that includes onions, leeks, chives, scallions, and shallots. It is grown, harvested and cured. The bulbs form cloves. Naked stalks climb out of the ground, and sometimes, but not always, white flowers form at the tops of these stems. You can harvest it from either the bulb or green shoots — both provide the flavor that you are seeking.

It has been grown for thousands of years all over the world. Horticulturalists say there are dozens, perhaps even hundreds, of varieties of garlic and there are estimates ranging from a low of 30 to a high of 300 separate strains. Each one offers a unique virtue, but the same flavor and healthful properties are common to all of these strains — the important thing is that it *is* garlic.

Nothing can quite compare with the taste of it.

"The flavor of fresh garlic has not, as yet, been duplicated by any processing techniques that I know of. Because garlic oxidizes so readily when it is cut, commercial products must add other substances such as citric acid and/or oil to preserve them. This alters the wonderfully distinctive flavor of garlic," writes Lloyd John Harris in his book *The Official Garlic Lovers Handbook* (published by Aris Books, of Berkeley, California, $7.95).

Grocery stores offer a wide variety of very good, whole clove garlics. Those little cardboard boxes with the clear windows in the center of the carton contain the real thing. When you cook with this, be sure to use all of any single clove you peel and open — it just doesn't keep fresh once it has been exposed to the air.

6

Growing Your Own..

Garlic is quite remarkably easy for you to cultivate on your own. If you do decide to go that route — ask the advice of any gardener or nurseryman and follow his instructions faithfully — remember that the "fresh" garlic label rarely means that it has just come straight out of the ground. While you *can* eat freshly pulled garlic, it is actually the drying and curing process that gives it its full and truly distinctive flavor.

Because it is cured, it retains its flavor and goodness for many months if you store it properly, again according to the directions. The key to a long shelf life for garlic is leaving it where air can circulate freely around it. Keep it in a cool and dry place — basements and garages are ideal.

You can braid garlic stems to form bunches that are pleasing to the eye, or you can store them in the types of mesh bags in which you usually find onions, in old nylon stockings or on wire racks.

Other storage methods include dehydrating, pureeing, marinating in vegetable or olive oil and refrigerating. Ironically, of all the storage options, placing whole cloves in the refrigerator is the least effective method of storage. It certainly works, but refrigerators tend to be a tad too damp and cold for ideal, long-term preservation. So if you store garlic in those little compartments on the door of the fridge, be sure you're going to use it fast unless you want to throw a lot of it away.

..And Curing It

If you grow garlic at home, dry the bulbs thoroughly for about two weeks in a closet or in the garage or basement. To cure them, trim the roots off, leaving about a half inch of stem, then braid or tie the bulbs together in bunches and hang them from rafters or herb drying stands for two weeks to a month. After that they are ready to eat, and if you have more than you can conveniently consume in short order, you can prepare it for longer-term storage.

Horticulturist and writer Susan Chamberlin tells how to do that in *The Official Garlic Lover's Handbook*. To puree, peel and run through a blender or food processor. Put the puree in a jar and add a teaspoon of lemon juice or some olive oil for each half pint of puree. Refrigerate for at least a day before opening the jar.

To dehydrate, slice the cloves into ⅛-inch slices and lay them out on a cheese cloth to dry in the sun. You can also use a gas oven. Leave them until they turn into little chips that snap. Then you can store them inside a tightly sealed jar in a cool cupboard for years. Do not refrigerate. Use them in soups, salads and sauces.

To marinate, slice and place in a jar of extra virgin olive oil in the refrigerator. You may add herbs if you wish. It is important to use extra virgin grade olive oil, even though it is more expensive, because lesser grades will congeal under refrigeration.

Garlic's Noble Past

The great medieval king, Charlemagne, ordered all of his subjects to grow garlic in their gardens, declaring it one of those rare herbs that are, "the friend of physicians and the praise of cooks..."

But the use of garlic goes far further back in history than the days of Charlemagne. Historians say that garlic receives mention in the earliest texts of recorded history, and played important roles in the cultures of the great nations of antiquity that flourished around the Mediterranean, such as Mesopotamia, Sumeria, Assyria, Egypt and Persia, as well as India and China.

Researchers have found references to garlic in Chinese texts dating back as far as 2,000 years before Christ walked the earth, which means that civilization has been familiar with garlic and its uses as a foodstuff and healing agent for at least 4,000 years.

Interestingly, the ancient Chinese thought garlic was especially good for purifying water and preventing food poisoning from improperly prepared meat and fish. That usage is confirmed by modern scientific findings which have shown that the germ killing properties in garlic can preserve meat, keeping it fresh and edible two to four times longer than meat untreated with garlic.

Yale University scholars have recently unearthed Babylonian tablets from the year 1,700 B.C. — almost 4,000 years ago — listing recipes that strongly feature garlic and onions.

Archeologists have found illustrations of a garlic clove in the tomb of the pharaoh, Tutankhamen.

Today, garlic grows in all regions of the world but nobody is quite sure where it originated precisely because it has been so popular in so many places for so many years.

Many historians suspect that garlic first took root, so to speak, some place in Asia — maybe Siberia — and was brought through

Asia minor to the Fertile Crescent, the Red Sea and the regions surrounding the fertile delta of the River Nile. From there it was probably spread to Europe by seagoing traders, and the rest, as they say, truly is history.

The Talmud

According to the *Talmud*, the authority on Jewish law and tradition, the eating of garlic satisfied hunger, kept the body warm, brightened the complexion, killed parasites in the body, removed jealousy and promoted love. Interestingly, the *Talmud* recommends garlic as an aphrodisiac and suggests eating it on Friday — the night set aside for marital love-making, according to garlic chronicler, Alexandra Hicks.

In ancient Greece, Hippocrates, the "father of modern medicine," used garlic for treating infections, wounds and intestinal disorders — not to mention a reportedly mean lamb stew and an outstanding vegetable soup. Roman legionnaires attributed their strength, courage and stamina to garlic and took it with them as they conquered their world — and thus spreading its use and cultivation everywhere they went.

Since then, garlic has enjoyed a huge importance in the cooking and cultures of Mediterranean countries such as Italy, Spain, Turkey, and on the North African coast, Morocco and Tunisia.

Curiously enough, in England and eventually in America, there was quite a bit of resistance to garlic, but the bulb has finally, and smashingly, made it big in the U.S.A. Look at the numbers: over 200 million pounds of garlic are grown commercially in this country every year.

And there is more.

It may strike you as somewhat strange, but there is even evidence to indicate that garlic has been given a demi-god status and worshipped — as well as being denounced as a demon — at a number of periods in history. I am not suggesting for a moment that we should take our enthusiasm for garlic to that kind of length but it does emphasize the intense effect garlic can have on people's hearts, minds and palates!

Let's take a closer look at the myths, or superstitions, if you will, because a startling amount of these are being confirmed scientifically today.

The Ancient World

The world still marvels today at the pyramids at Giza, built by the ancient Egyptians as a stunning monument to their ingenuity and their kings. Inscriptions inside these structures in the Valley of the Kings indicate that the workers who built them subsisted largely on onions, garlic and radishes, and that to them they were more than mere foodstuffs.

The Egyptians actually credited these foods, especially garlic, with magical and medicinal powers responsible for the physical stamina and spiritual integrity necessary for the workers to complete their tasks. And apparently the workers subscribed to the same theory, because when the supplies of garlic ran out, they went on strike — something certainly almost previously unheard of in that day and age.

An Egyptian holy book, the *Codex Ebers*, was discovered in 1878 by the distinguished German archaeologist George Ebers. It dates from about 1550 B.C. and lists more than 800 therapeutic formulas in use at the time; 22 of them were based on garlic and these were said to heal headaches, heart problems, body weakness, human bites, intestinal parasites, throat tumors, and solve any problems relating to childbirth and the menstrual cycle.

The Bible tells how the ancient Jews considered garlic to be a magic talisman against evil spirits, protecting people from the contagion and epidemic disease brought on by angry demons.

In ancient Palestine, garlic was believed to promote fertility in women having difficulty conceiving children and it was also firmly recommended as protection against the "Evil Eye" — just as, many centuries later, it was reported to protect against vampires and werewolves.

The prophet of Islam, Mohammed, recommended garlic as an antidote to the stings and bites of poisonous insects, snakes and other animals.

Classical Greece

The ancient Greeks used garlic talismans to guard against the mischief of the *Neriades*, malicious, beautiful half-divine, half-human nymphs who tried to lead wives and mothers-to-be astray.

Throughout the civilizations of ancient Rome, early India, and

China, garlic was considered potent medicine, as it was through-out Medieval Europe.

And on into what we now consider modern times, garlic has maintained its place as a favorite food and valued medicine. In particular, in the south of France (in a region called Provence, where the ancient city of Avignon is located); in Italy and in Spain, garlic assumed a profound and fundamental importance in cooking and medicine.

Remember Dracula!

The strangest belief about garlic originated in Eastern Europe, where people used it to repel vampires. We may chuckle at the notion now, but these people were not fooling around and it wasn't all that long ago that they lived in mortal fear that their life blood would be sucked from them as they slept.

To them, vampires were a very serious business indeed, and the most effective protection against them was garlic. They hung garlands of garlic around their necks, and in bunches in the doorways and windows of their homes to keep them safe.

They also believed that once they caught a vampire and killed it, garlic could help keep it dead — hence the literary tradition, carried on in countless Hollywood horror flicks, of stuffing garlic in a vampire's mouth and filling its coffin with whole cloves before burial (this, of course, presupposes catching the vampire and killing it either with a silver bullet or burying a stake in its heart).

Native Americana

American Indians used garlic as a charm to rid young maidens of unwanted suitors. South American revolutionary San Martin, who led the fights for independence of Argentina, Chile and Peru in the 19th century made his men, horses and mules, sniff and chew garlic to combat altitude sickness as they crossed the towering Andes mountain range.

Cuba

In Cuba, 13 cloves of garlic at the end of a string worn around the neck for a period of 13 days, no more, no less, is regarded as a sure-fire way to keep jaundice away. For maximum effectiveness, arise in the middle of the night of the thirteenth day, says the tradition, go to the intersection of two streets, take off the garlic necklace, fling it behind you and run home without looking back. If you did look over your shoulder, said the tradition, a boogey man would hunt you down.

Food For The Masses

Lloyd J. Harris, author of *The Book of Garlic* (from the Addison-Wesley Publishing Co., $11.95) says the history of garlic makes one point abundantly clear "...that garlic has always been a 'peoples' food and remedy (magical and medical); and where the people loved it most, the upper classes (priests, kings and aristocrats, politicians) created taboos against it. The people worshipped it anyway."

Garlic Festivals

For many thousands of years the people of the world have celebrated garlic with feasting, (in which garlic and garlic enhanced dishes featured prominently, of course) festival and celebration. Now we do it all over America as well, although without any question California is the garlic-festival capital.

There is of course, the daddy of them all, the Gilroy Garlic Festival, which is the center of the garlic industry in the country. It began in 1978 and is held, complete with food booths, a golf tournament, and all kinds of contests and exhibitions, on the last weekend of July each year. For more information write to: Gilroy Garlic Festival, PO Box 2311, Gilroy, CA 95020.

The Berkeley Garlic Festival, Berkeley, California, is held in mid-July each year. It is sponsored by the *Lovers of the Stinking Rose*, and The Berkeley Garlic Festival Committee, and upwards of fifty local restaurants feature garlic on their nightly dinner menus for two weeks. The special events include a film festival, and a 'garlic dance'. For information write: Lovers of the Stinking Rose, 1621 Fifth Street, Berkeley, CA 94710.

The annual Garlic Fest, in Covington, Kentucky, is held every February, and features recipe cook offs, a bulb peeling contest and a Miss Garlic beauty pageant. For information write: Coving Haus, 100 West Sixth Street, Covington, KY 41011.

The Fitchburg Garlic Festival is held at an Italian church, Madonna of the Holy Rosary, in Fitchburg, Massachusetts, every June. For information write Rev. Pat Biscardi.

3 The Great Healer

Here's where we go beyond mere character and ancestry to delve into the reasons why we can truly apply the term "wonder food" to garlic.

Healing power, medicinal value, a cure for what ails you, call it what you want, garlic is the real thing.

"Thousands of years of folklore couldn't all be wrong and laboratory analysis has proven that it is true," says Dr. Victor Gurewich, director of the Tufts University Vascular Laboratory, at St. Elizabeth's Hospital, in Boston. He and his colleagues conducted extensive tests on garlic and onions which showed garlic has an amazing ability to lower total cholesterol and confer protection against heart attacks and hardening of the arteries in several other ways.

Scientific understanding of the natural gift of garlic has come a long way in less than a century. Around the year 1900, garlic ointments, compresses and compounds were the common treatment of choice. Military surgeons in World War I, who did not have modern antibiotics available to them, used it to cleanse wounds, combat infections and prevent and treat gangrene. It worked so well that British surgeons still relied on it extensively during World War II, even though antibiotics were available by then.

Even today in the Soviet Union, garlic is still used to kill bacteria and fight infections, and some tests show it is more effective than antibiotics for specific types of bacterial infection termed "gram negative." Throughout Europe this has earned garlic the nickname "Russian penicillin."

Since the 1940s, scientific investigation has proven garlic possesses a stunning array of medicinal properties. Investigators say that it:

- Acts as an antiseptic
- Fights infection
- Contains chemicals which prevent cancer
- Thins the blood, reducing clotting in high risk heart patients
- Lowers the blood pressure
- Reduces cholesterol
- Controls triglycerides
- Stimulates the immune system
- Prevents and relieves chronic bronchitis
- Acts as a decongestant and expectorant

The National Library of Medicine, in Bethesda, Maryland, contains over 125 scientific papers written about the medicinal value of garlic since 1983 alone. And in most cases, say noted physicians, you can eat a clove or two a day, cut up in salads and soups, and derive the same level of protection.

Garlic has an amazingly high sulphur content, and it is this, experts say, that makes all the difference.

Let's examine some of these findings in greater detail.

Heart Disease

Heart disease is the leading killer of Americans, accounting for nearly one in two deaths in this country every year. Garlic can reduce those numbers and protect you and your family. That's good news.

Garlic can prevent heart attacks and strokes by controlling the key variables of high cholesterol, high triglycerides, high blood pressure and atherosclerosis — the deadly process of plaque formation and fat deposits inside the arteries. These factors create blockages in the circulatory system that ultimately can choke blood flow to the heart muscle or brain.

The simplest explanation is that garlic thins the blood. Dr. George Blodgett spent six years doing laboratory research back in the 1920s and saw microscopic evidence of garlic's workings. "It dissolves fat particles and out-of-place blood clots and keeps them in suspension until they can be eliminated through the bowel — as long as it's circulating and your body's excreting it, it can't hurt you. The stuff works, and it beats me why we insist on fancier, more expensive prescription medicines when nature already provides what we need."

He used garlic as a heart medication during his nearly 70-year practice because it worked. That's all he cared about. "What else do you need to know?"

An esteemed German physician, Dr. Hans Reuter, of Cologne, Germany, reported clinical studies in the mid-to-late 1970s proving the effectiveness of garlic against heart disease on three fronts: In controlling cholesterol, blood pressure and fatty deposits in the arteries. He recommended one to three cloves daily, that's all. Simply add them to soup or salad.

But modern medicine works in mysterious ways, and for reasons not readily apparent it is highly resistant to change. Conservatism and caution seems built into the profession. With rare exceptions physicians have been highly skeptical of Dr. Reuter's findings, despite his high standing in the academic community.

Lowering Cholesterol

Investigators in India, Bulgaria, Libya and Japan have produced some powerful scientific evidence supporting garlic's role in warding off heart disease. American scientists, I'm afraid to say, tend to be insular to say the least — some critics might say self centered and egotistical — and look down their noses at any work carried out by scientists other than American scientists.

They also discount what they dismiss as anecdotal reports or empirical evidence — such as the seventy years of case histories that Dr. Blodgett could produce. Unless the evidence comes from what are called controlled, scientific trials, they insist, such reports simply don't count.

Happily, a few suspected that where there was smoke there might well be fire.

One of them was Dr. David Kritchevsky, now associate director of the Wistar Institute in Philadelphia.

"I was doing postdoctoral work in Switzerland," he says, "when I discovered that my landlady — a 66-year-old woman who looked 44 and acted 22 — attributed her good health to the fact that she ate a clove of garlic chopped up in her salad every single night."

He was inclined at first to dismiss her report as superstitious nonsense, but he discovered that other Europeans offered similar witness. That prompted him to begin a serious investigation into garlic's possible impact on heart disease.

His experiments demonstrated that rabbits fed a diet which included garlic oil had 10 percent lower blood cholesterol levels, and from a low of 15 to a high of 45 percent less fat in their arteries than rabbits which did not consume the garlic oil. Subsequent studies confirmed that the effect held true in rats as well.

Armed with this evidence, Kritchevsky then reviewed scientific literature from around the world and finally concluded that garlic does exactly what his landlady claimed. But he still had reservations. "The trouble is, the dosage required for humans seems pretty high."

Other studies have laid his fears to rest.

Results from India

The prestigious British medical journal *The Lancet* published a study by two Indian cardiologists which showed that raw garlic will indeed protect you from heart disease.

You don't have to change anything else in your diet, mind you, all you have to do is add garlic. Of course, the greater care you take to observe a low-fat, and high-fiber diet, the better off you will be. But Drs. Bordia and Bansal, of the Department of Medicine at R.N.T. Medical College in Udaipur, India, found that garlic controls cholesterol so effectively that it even overcomes the cardiotoxic effects of butter fat.

In their controlled experiments they gave their subjects a meal that included a quarter pound serving of butter. Just as they expected, blood cholesterol levels soared. Then they repeated the experiment, but this time they added 50 grams of raw garlic to the butter (equal to about two cloves). The results were truly astonishing. The garlic lowered blood cholesterol by more than 25 percent from the pre-meal fasting level.

Even after consuming that very large, highly imprudent, amount of butter, the addition of garlic had left these patients better off than before they had eaten. The garlic also counteracted a tendency for blood to clot in unwanted ways after a high fat meal.

The authors wrote, "It is obvious that garlic has a very significant protective action against hyperlipidaemia (high cholesterol) and blood-coagulation changes, which are normal after fat ingestion." And all this without the high cost and high risk of the prescription drugs that are so frequently used to lower cholesterol. The report continued: "Clinically, garlic could avoid most of these drawbacks and could be recommended for long-term use without any danger of toxicity. It would be particularly useful in preventing alimentary hyperlipidaemia in persons who do not have manifest signs of arteriosclerosis but are predisposed on account of diabetes, hypertension, family history of stroke and heart disease." And that means, all told, about 170 million Americans.

New Studies

Studies published in the *American Journal of Clinical Nutrition* verify these findings.

Other human tests showed that about one-eighth of a cup of fresh garlic juice every day achieved a drastic drop in blood cholesterol, from an average reading of 305 to 218 in two months.

Still other studies show garlic has an amazing ability to discriminate between "good" HDL and "bad" LDL cholesterol and do the right thing by you. LDL increases heart disease risk by promoting fat deposits inside the arteries; they are, fuguratively, dump-trucks in your blood which drop loads of fat along the inside walls of your arteries. HDL is just the opposite and protects you; it is, figuratively, an earth mover, scooping loads of fat from inside your arteries and hauling it away to the liver and bowel where it can be eliminated.

"We found that garlic or onions in amounts that you'd consider normal to eat, raised the level of HDL cholesterol just as effectively as daily, vigorous exercise," says Dr. Victor Gurewich, of Tufts University in Massachusetts.

Dr. Myung Chi, of Lincoln University, in Missouri, has confirmed this effect of garlic in his own experiments and believes it may also prove effective in relieving high blood pressure.

Garlic Concentrate

Those incredibly innovative Japanese are coming up with something clever and new every day. And the field of garlic is no different to them, it appears, than the world of automobiles or electronics. They have developed a garlic extract concentrate which eliminates that bothersome odor while retaining all of these wonderfully beneficial properties. They call it *Kyolic*. And it works.

In 1987, Dr. Benjamin Lau at Loma Linda University, in California, used Kyolic in a heart disease experiment with dramatic effect. They found that a gram of Kyolic (the equivalent of about nine cloves of garlic) lowered total cholesterol about ten percent on average, but as much as 50 percent in some individuals, and lowered LDL cholesterol levels in 70 percent of the volunteers in the study.

Clot Busters..

Garlic actually dissolves life threatening blood clots. Dr. Martyn Bailey, of Georgetown University, in Washington D.C. has produced laboratory evidence that a chemical in garlic, called adenosine, blocks the production of a blood compound named fibronolytic, which makes blood sticky and causes clotting.

To put it another way, this means that garlic thins the blood. And adenosine isn't the only weapon in garlic's arsenal, says chemistry professor Dr. Eric Block, of the State University of New York. By teaming adenosine with a chemical Dr. Block discovered called ajoene (which is what you'd call a medical marvel, because it also has antibiotic properties and promotes wound healing), garlic can give untimely blood clots a knock out punch.

Block says quite bluntly that, "As an antithrombotic agent (clot buster), ajoene is at least as potent as aspirin." And aspirin has been recognized as one of the most effective anticoagulants, or blood thinners, going. His animal experiments show that a single dose of ajoene will shut down platelet aggregation (unwanted clotting) by 100 percent and keep it that way for 24 hours.

All of these researchers stress quite firmly that garlic has absolutely no side effects of any kind. The only risk you can possibly run as a confirmed consumer of garlic is that of offending your friends. Kyolic can eliminate that hazard if it concerns you.

But that's just the tip of the iceberg when it comes to the healing powers of garlic.

Infection Fighter

Garlic kills germs. In 1944, chemist Chester Cavallito identified the smelly compound in garlic, called allicin, and demonstrated that it was a highly effective antibiotic. Other tests have confirmed that garlic is an even more powerful germ killer than either penicillin or tetracycline.

The list of microbes that garlic can slay includes botulism, tuberculosis, diarrhea, staph, dysentery, pneumonia, sepsis and typhoid. Reports list 72 seperate bugs garlic can bump off: bacteria, yeast, fungus (tuberculosis is the best-known fungal infection) parasites and protozoa all yield to garlic.

Cooking neutralizes allicin, so you need raw garlic for its antibiotic properties. Many doctors will tell you that a compress of mashed garlic can keep cuts and wounds clean and free of infection.

There are some reports that applying garlic directly to skin cancers makes the tumor disappear within weeks.

Virus Fighter

The most significant recent discovery is that garlic also kills viruses. This has potentially enormous significance.

It means that the next time you feel a cold or flu coming on, add a few cloves of raw garlic to your chicken soup and you'll not only feel better for a while, you'll beat the illness outright.

"If you do it early enough, you may not even get sick," says Dr. James North, chief of microbiology at Brigham Young University, in Provo, Utah.

He conducted experiments showing garlic as a potent virus killer, and the implications of his findings are stunning. Not only do common ailments such as the cold come within garlic's medicinal reach, but more serious diseases such as herpes, polio and, dare we say it?, even AIDS may succumb.

His data show garlic extract kills with near 100 percent effectiveness:

- Human rhinovirus, which causes colds

- Parainfluenza 3, a common flu and respiratory virus

- Herpes simplex 1, which causes fever blisters

- Herpes simplex 2, responsible for genital herpes

In addition, garlic has killed the polio virus with 90 percent effectiveness and proven capable of tackling the deadly HIV or AIDS virus. Once scientists identify the active virus-killing chemical in garlic, they may be able to make a concentrated pill for treating these very serious ailments.

Cancer

Now hear this: nobody is saying garlic cures cancer. The reason I'm stating that is because the American Cancer Society hunts people down who use the word *cure* in connection with cancer as if they were witches. Having said that, let's take a look at the evidence that garlic's healing touch extends even to the " Big C."

As long ago as 1952, Russian scientists were using garlic extracts against human tumors. Colon cancer — one of the most common forms of the disease — may be particularly susceptible to the power of garlic.

Dr. Michael Wargovich, of the University of Texas, M.D. Anderson Hospital and Tumor Institute, has found that mice treated with a chemical in garlic are 75 percent less likely to develop malignancies in the large bowel. The National Cancer Institute is taking these findings seriously enough to investigate the matter further and currently places garlic extremely high on its list of "chemopreventives," or substances that block carcinogens.

Bladder cancer may not stand a chance against it, either. Animal experiments by Dr. Benjamin Lau, of Loma Linda University in California, demonstrated that garlic extract (Kyolic) inhibited this deadly malignancy.

Chinese researchers, together with scientists at Cornell University and the National Cancer Institute, say garlic, as well as onions and scallions, can dramatically cut your risk of stomach cancer. The more you eat, the lower your risk, and depending on how much you are prepared to eat, you can almost triple your protection.

Diabetes

The U.S. Department of Agriculture's Human Nutrition Center, in Beltsville, Maryland has demonstrated that the herb can reduce not only levels of blood fat, but blood sugar too, at the same time increasing the level of insulin in the blood. That spells one thing: better diabetes control.

Dr. Tarig Abdullah of the Akbar Clinic and Research Institute, in Panama City, Florida, has produced dramatic evidence that garlic revs up the body's immune system.

He and nine other volunteers ate either raw garlic or Kyolic extract. He then drew the volunteers' blood and the blood of a control group of people who had not eaten any garlic at all. The next step was to extract key immune system components such as white blood cells and killer cells (a type of white blood cell that attacks and kills invaders). They were mixed in a lab dish with cancer cells. The result was astonishing — killer cells from the garlic eaters destroyed from 140 to 160 percent more cancer cells than did blood from the non-garlic eaters.

Abdullah ate large amounts, 10 to 15 cloves a day, but is convinced you can obtain a protective effect from smaller doses. He also believes his finding may be of extreme importance to AIDS treatment. On a more casual note, he reports eating a couple of raw garlic cloves every day and says that as a result he has not had a cold since he started the habit in 1973.

Better Living, (Naturally)

The chemical breakdown of garlic provides some real insight into its many medicinal talents. It is a mineral and vitamin rich food, but it is the especially high concentration of sulphur compounds (allyl sulphides) that truly set it apart.

According to analysis by the U.S. Department of Agriculture, a single clove of garlic contains:

- Seven calories
- .31 grams (gm) of protein
- .01 gm fat
- 1.5 gm carbohydrate
- 1.4 milligrams (mg) of calcium
- 10 mg phosphorus
- .07 mg iron
- .9 mg sodium
- 26 mg potassium
- .01 mg B1
- .004 mg B2
- .02 mg niacin
- .75 mg. C

The Healing Ingredients

Alliin, Allicin and Allinase by name are the big three for you to particularly remember. These are sulphur compounds. They have drawn the attention of serious scientists since the illustrious Louis Pasteur pointed to the antiseptic properties of garlic in 1858.

In the 1940s, Dr. Arthur Stoll, a Nobel Prize-winning scientist, uncovered alliin, which he showed to be the "parent" compound of the germ fighting process. It must be broken down before garlic gives off its characteristic odor and before it turns into an antibiotic. The enyzme allinase, also present in garlic, starts the reaction. All it takes is cutting or crushing the garlic clove and the two combine, to produce allicin. For the science buffs among you, the technical name is allylthiosulphinic acid diallyl disulphide. This in turns breaks diallyl disulphide (the stinky stuff) and allythiosulphinate, the medicinal essence.

Even though standard antibiotics are a bit stronger than what garlic provides, U.S. researchers have noted that garlic is more effective against certain germs called gram-negative organisms, than conventional medications.

Selenium and Germanium

Garlic is loaded with selenium, an important trace element, and Dr. Gerhard Schrauzer of the University of California at San Diego, says it offers protection against cancer, atherosclerosis and normalizes blood pressure. It is also an anti-oxidant, a chemical that neutralizes harsh compounds called free-radicals which accelerate the aging process, so this may account for the anti-aging power of garlic.

Germanium is a relatively recent discovery — like selenium, it is also a trace element — and it is thought to offer significant health benefits because it stimulates oxygen circulation throughout the human body. Garlic contains this trace element too.

And More...

Even more evidence of garlic's entry into modern medicine and nutrition is clear. Dr. William Castelli, director of the world's famous Framingham Study on cholesterol and heart disease, includes garlic on his list of foods that contribute to the prevention of heart disease.

It seems as if almost every day there is a new study on garlic mentioned in the media. I've given up trying to keep up with it all, writes Lloyd John Harris in his *The Official Garlic Lovers Handbook*. What's encouraging for those who believe in garlic's healing benefits, he says, is that more and more of the studies mentioned in the press are by American researchers.

So why has the U.S. medical establishment shown such a low level of interest in medicinal uses of garlic? The answer is probably an economic one. The costs of establishing the efficacy and safety of any new pharmaceutical are quite high. Yet, there is little profit to be made in marketing a folk remedy that people can obtain quite cheaply and administer to themselves.

Ross S. Feldberg, Ph.D
Associate Professor of Biology
Tufts University

There's More

And there is a legion of everyday complaints for which garlic can also provide the answer. It can be used for pain of all kinds mashed, as a tincture, or as an oil, on wounds, abscesses or on stubborn skin infections, although it is strong and those with sensitive skins should be careful. It can cause blistering.

It is also effective as a garlic and water enema in effecting a speedy recovery from amoebic dysentry, and is used widely in Mexico and in the countries of Central America.

The prominent natural medicine authority, Dr. Dian Dincin Buchman, in her book *Herbal Medicine* recommends a garlic syrup for asthma, which has been in her family for many years.

The dosage is one teaspoon with or without water every 15 minutes until the spasm is controlled. Afterwards give the patient one teaspoon every two to three hours for the rest of the day.

The recipe: ½ pound peeled garlic buds; equal amounts vinegar and distilled water to cover the buds; half pint glycerine; 1½ pounds of honey.

Put peeled garlic, vinegar and water in a wide-mouth jar, close tighly and shake well. Let it stand in a cool place for four or five days, shaking twice daily. Add the glycerine, shake the jar and let stand one more day. Strain and blend in the honey. Store in a cool place.

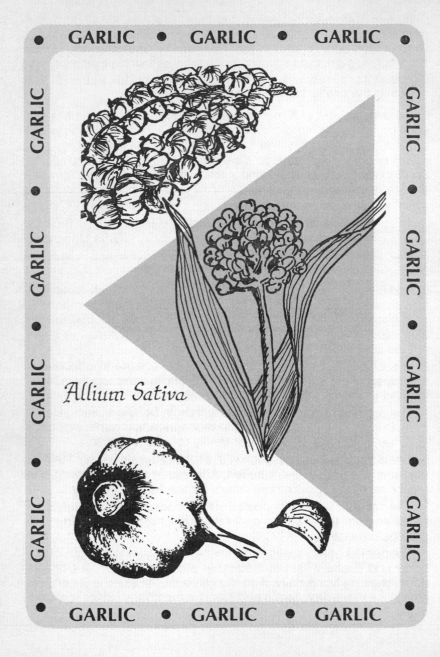

Allium Sativa

4 "Green" Garlic

Festivals to celebrate, newsletters to propagate the good word, uses in gardening, pet care, and other applications are things you might never have imagined about garlic.

"Green" does not refer to the color of the bulb (although it can be green) but rather to garlic's environmental friendliness. It is a great alternative insecticide, capable of ridding houses, gardens, lawns, farms, pets and trees of pests without the harshness and toxicity of chemicals and without adding more damage to an already burdened environment.

The issue of "Green Consumerism" is going to be one of the biggest and most pressing issues of the 1990s, according to environmentalists the world over. Our relentless use of plastics and other throwaway materials, the endless stockpiling of refuse and waste materials and the reliance on chemicals for everything from washing floors to fueling rockets is quite literally endangering the existence of our planet.

Huge forests in Europe and North America are withering, lakes are dying and weather is changing in ways scientists don't understand, but which they believe relate to the pollution of the earth.

We can wage war for the earth's survival in tiny ways every day in our own homes and daily lives; with the products we buy, with the packaging we insist on and with the compounds we choose for what seem to be the most simple of tasks.

Believe it or not, the insect repellants we use around our homes contribute to overall pollution. And if we choose safe alternatives, we can make a very real difference in the struggle to preserve the environment.

It is into this large scenario that garlic can make at least a cameo appearance.

No one claims that garlic can solve the pollution crisis single-handedly; its ability to change the chemical composition of the atmosphere may not be as dramatic as its talent for changing your internal chemistry, but every little bit helps. That's the point organizations such as Greenpeace and Earth Watch are trying to make.

Better Than D.D.T.

Garlic kills bugs dead. The difference is that garlic won't hurt people, the soil, the water or the air. Mosquitoes, including those carrying yellow fever and encephalitis, drop dead in its presence.

The U.S. and other nations have phased out D.D.T. because of the health horrors it can cause. Instead of seeking natural alternatives, the pros have gone out in search of "safe" chemicals. The new pesticides are organo-phosphorous compounds and the Journal of the American Medical Association has stated that while they don't stay in the environment — or the human body — as long as D.D.T., they are much more poisonous.

Well, in its small way, garlic can help you avoid exposure to these horrid compounds. Many studies have shown that it can act as an effective, safe and inexpensive shoo-fly-don't-bother-me agent.

David Greenstock, vice-chairman of The Henry Doubleday Research Association in England, has produced a garlic emulsion that kills malarial mosquitoes that have developed an immunity to D.D.T. Here are some "kill" figures to show how garlic solvents work against other pests:

- 87 percent of fireworm infestation
- 83 percent of cockchafer larvae
- 91 percent of mole crickets
- 82 percent of grey field slugs
- 95 percent of onion fly larvae
- 98 percent of cabbage white caterpillars
- 98 percent of ermine moth caterpillars

A laboratory experiment produced some especially admirable

results against the pea weevil, killing 87 percent of them, L. John Harris reports in *The Book of Garlic*. This is an insect related to the boll weevil, known to decimate cotton crops, and which many American growers claim requires D.D.T.

Greenstock has clearly demonstrated that while garlic "kills bugs dead," it is completely safe and harmless to livestock and wildlife and birds. If anything, veterinarians believe garlic improves the health of animals.

Organic Gardening With Garlic

For these reasons, it is standard practice for organic gardeners today to border their plantings with rows of garlic and spray their crops with a garlic solution.

The same should go for you at home: If you are growing just a few herbs or a few tomatoes, or are raising a more extensive vegetable garden or an orchard of fruit trees, plant some garlic in amongst your crops, horticulturalists recommend. It will repel the pests and leave you with something else tasty to eat at the end of the growing season — not a heightened risk of cancer some time in the future, which is a real threat from some chemical sprays.

How to Make a Safe Bug Spray

The same mechanisms in garlic that kill germs in people also seem to hit insects hard and keep them away from plants. Some researchers say garlic can inhibit protein synthesis in larvae, killing them. Others say it suppresses the respiratory metabolism.

Here is David Greenstock's formula, as reported by John Harris, publisher of Aris Books:

"Take three ounces of chopped garlic and let soak in two teaspoons (50 cc) of mineral oil for 24 hours. Then slowly add a pint of water in which ¼-ounce of oil-based soap (Palmolive) has been dissolved, and stir well. Strain liquid through fine gauze and store in china or glass container to prevent a reaction with metals. Use it in a dilution of one part to 20 of water to begin with, then one to 100 thereafter. Apply to plants as spray."

This is a simple preparation, effective and non-toxic. My wife and I have used it, and we saved a maple sapling from certain death by caterpillar and aphid infestation.

Flea Repellant

What's good for the garden is good for pets. If you can successfully feed your dog, cat or other pet a single clove of garlic a day, you will effectively control the parasitic population in the animal's coat without resorting to harsh sprays, powders or shampoos.

The simplest way to do this is chop up a clove and mix it in with daily chow. It's unlikely that an animal will chew a whole clove, plain, but with animals, anything is possible. If you mix it in with the daily meal, however, you eliminate the problem of finicky, furry friends.

Here are other things, of a more pedestrian nature, you should know about garlic.

Garlic Capital

Gilroy, California, bills itself as the "Garlic Capital of the World." It boasts a $54 million a year garlic industry in a town with a population of only 27,400.

Humorist Will Rogers described Gilroy as, "the only town in America where you can marinate a steak by hanging it on the clothesline," in reference to the pungent odor that pervades the city.

Obviously, making as much money every year out of garlic as the residents of Gilroy do, they're laughing at jokes like that all the way to the bank. With that kind of income, they've got nothing to be ashamed of compared to their economic big brother, the famous "Silicon Valley," several dozen miles to the north where a major center of the U.S. computer industry is located.

Ninety percent of the garlic consumed in the 50 states is shipped through Gilroy for processing and packaging, much of it grown within a radius of 90 miles of the town.

The Gilroy-based Fresh Garlic Association reports that Americans gobble 24 ounces of whole garlic per person each year. That's the equivalent of about 20 bulbs per capita, or 5 billion heads a year!

The good folks in Gilroy have written a book called *The Complete Garlic Lover's Cookbook* (published by Celestial Art Books, Berkeley, California, $19.95). It includes recipes and practical pointers on how to spot, treat and eat garlic the right way.

Fresh garlic may vary in color from creamy white to slightly purplish, but it should be plump and firm, not spongy, soft or shriveled up.

If you're going for processed forms of garlic, make sure they come in tightly sealed containers.

Storage

The Gilroy garlic experts say the best way to store the bulb is in a cool, dry place with plenty of ventilation, and they warn against storing it in the refrigerator unless first immersed in oil.

The longer you store garlic in the open air, the milder it will be when you finally use it, but by all means use it. The bulb may even develop some sprouts as it sits; don't let those put you off.

Store garlic powders or other dehydrated forms away from the stove and windows with direct sunlight streaming in — heat and light can knock the natural flavor out of processed garlic in pretty short order.

Keep an Eye Peeled

Here are the correct techniques for peeling garlic: If you only want to use a few cloves, press them between the thumb and forefinger to loosen the skin first, then place on a cutting board and press down on them with the flat side of a heavy kitchen knife.

For larger quantities, drop cloves into boiling water for a single minute and drain and then they'll peel easily. Five seconds in a microwave oven achieves the same effect.

Please note, peeling is not always mandatory. You can try cooking unpeeled cloves in a hot pan; this will protect the garlic meat from burning, and the skin will slip off when the garlic is soft. And if you're going to cook the garlic in a soup or stew, why bother going to the trouble of peeling? The flavor will reach the dish and you can either throw out the garlic later or press the soft garlic out of the skin with your knife and fork while you're eating.

Counteracting the Odor

There are techniques to contain the fragrance left on your hands after peeling and chopping. Try wearing rubber gloves while you're working. If that doesn't suit you, rub your fingers with salt and lemon juice afterward, then rinse with cold water.

The Gilroy garlic experts say the best solution they have found is to clasp their fingers around the bowl of a stainless steel teaspoon under running water for a few moments. There is a chemical reaction which takes place that does indeed eliminate the odor from the fingers.

Garlic odor on the breath is most easily controlled by eating fresh parsley. Parsley has been called "nature's mouthwash" by garlic lovers because of its effectiveness. Chewing on a coffee bean or two also seems to do the trick.

Common Varieties

The most common types grown commercially are probably related to these groups:

● *Late* garlic has a reputation for keeping a long time. The narrow, upright, dark green leaves and the white sheath surrounding the clove distinguish late garlic from other varieties. The clove ranges in color from light pink to deep red.

● *Early* garlic has broader leaves than the late type and they're light to pale green in color. This strain often displays purplish veins in the skin.

● *Creole* is common in Mexico and South America. The plant resembles the late garlic, except it is taller and lighter in color. The skin covering the cloves is dark pink.

● *Chileno* garlic is a variation on creole with larger cloves.

● *Chilean*, while obviously grown in South America, is also found in Japan, Formosa, India and Spain. The bulbs are white, flat and resemble a tangerine in shape and clove arrangement. The color of the cloves is dark pink to wine.

● *Egyptian* is tall and fast growing. It produces large, white bulbs which contain a lot of small cloves in white sheaths.

● *Elephant* garlic is an extremely mild form of garlic which has begun to find its way onto many supermarket shelves. The bulb is approximately the size of a tennis ball.

● *Italian* is grown in Louisiana and in other sub-tropical parts of the country. Its pink or purplish cloves are stronger in flavor and smaller than the *Creole* which is also grown in Louisiana. The garlic bulbs of this strain are not unlike the artichoke in appearance. The cloves, which are arranged just like artichoke leaves, have thin layered skins that comes off easily. This plant differs from the Creole in that it has lighter green leaves.

• *Silverskin* is the name given to many garlic strains which have that familiar white outer covering. This the basic white garlic that many nurseries will offer to the would be gardener cultivator. It grows strongly all across the country.

• *Spanish Rojo (Red)*. This powerfully flavored variety originated in Spain, hence the name. It is very tolerant to drought.

• *Rocambole*. Sometimes called *serpent garlic* because of the coiled shape of its looping green stems, the bulbs are smaller in size than plain garlic although they are equally as pungent. The baby bulbs that form after the flowers fade can be eaten fresh, and are delicious on salads, or they can be pickled.

How Much To Use

The Gilroy experts suggest starting with these amounts, which they admit are on the low side. As your tastes change, you may wish to add more:

For meats: use ⅛ to ¼ teaspoon of garlic powder or 1½ to 2 teaspoons of garlic salt or two to three cloves of fresh garlic for every two pounds of pork, beef, lamb or other meats you cook.

Sauces: use ⅛ to ¼ teaspoon of garlic powder or two cloves of fresh garlic for three cups of barbecue, tomato or other sauce.

Soups: for meat stock or vegetable soup add ⅛ teaspoon of garlic powder or two cloves of fresh garlic.

Pickled foods: add ⅛ to ¼ teaspoon of dehydrated, chopped or minced garlic, or two to three cloves fresh.

Relishes: add ⅛ teaspoon dehydrated minced garlic or two fresh cloves to two pints of chutney or relish.

5 Vinegar Power
Mineral Power

It is ironic that another common food item — vinegar — with a reputation among some for smelling odd could be so good for you. But it is true.

For optimum good health and longevity, the experts recommend a glass of water with two spoonsful of apple cider vinegar mixed in, at least twice a day. And they suggest that it is very much better to drink the potion once before every meal, every morning on awakening and before going to sleep at night. That is because there are 22 minerals essential for human health, and apple cider vinegar contains 19 of these minerals in exactly the right amounts.

The main benefits from this inexpensive health tonic (which costs less than a penny a day) is a strong and regular heart beat, a cast-iron digestive tract that nothing can disturb, a pair of kidneys that will never quit, and "freedom from all this allergy business," according to one enthusiastic doctor.

Now that sounds like a very good bargain indeed.

Shortly before his death, my friend Doctor Blodgett gave me a copy of his treasured book, *Folk Medicine, A Vermont Doctor's Guide to Good Health,* by D.C. Jarvis, M.D., which was first published by Henry Holt and Company in 1958.

Country Wisdom

The author, Dr. Jarvis, was a dyed-in-the-wool physician, ophthalmologist and otolaryngologist, as well as an enthusiast of the ways of folk medicine as they developed in the harsh and hauntingly beautiful climes of his native Vermont. In his own practice, he employed the methods that struck him as most sensible; those that worked stayed in his bag of tricks and those that were not effective, he discarded.

Much like Dr. Blodgett, Jarvis seemed more interested in helping people feel better than in simply marching in step with his medical brethren.

And, without any question, Dr. Jarvis was firmly convinced that taking simple apple cider vinegar could make any living thing — particularly men, women and children — healthier and more efficient. For everyone who sought a more enjoyable, lengthier, life, he said, it was a tonic that simply could not be ignored.

And it all boiled down to one very simple word...

Potassium

And that is because folk medicine practitioners, like Jarvis, believe that potassium is the most important of all of the minerals that are necessary for good health. "It is so essential to the life of every living thing that without it there would be no life," he wrote.

In the last five to ten years, orthodox medical researchers all over the world have proven the importance of potassium in a number of ways, thus endorsing the findings of the country doctor from New England. Dr. Louis Tobian, at the University of Minnesota School of Medicine, in Minneapolis, conducted a number of important experiments which clearly demonstrated that a proper potassium intake can dramatically reduce the symptoms in patients suffering from heart beat irregularities by well in excess of 50 percent, and will also insure that every single chemical reaction in the body works at its best. Other studies conducted in a number of centers have shown that nerve and muscle functions throughout the entire human body can suffer severely when the sodium-potassium balance is off.

One absolutely fundamental fact all doctors know today is that potassium counteracts the damaging effects of sodium and prevents high blood pressure. It stops unwanted fluid retention and regulates the body's water balance. It normalizes the heart rhythm, and works inside cells to keep sodium in check.

Dr. Tobian recommends eating a banana and a potato or grapefruit every day to make sure that you get all the potassium your body needs. And these are certainly good foods, and you should ensure they are a regular part of your daily diet. They are very low in fat and high in fiber. And they have so few calories that they can be eaten almost at will without worrying about weight gain.

And to get all of the potassium that ideally, your body should have every day, you cannot find a better source than vinegar, writes Jarvis — and apple cider vinegar is the best kind.

Dr. Blodgett believed "there is something" that occurs in the vinegar that makes the potassium more effective than if it comes from any other source. There are two reasons for that. First, other minerals in the vinegar activate and "potentiate" the potassium — that is to say they make it work better. Dr. Jarvis agrees.

He writes: "I have come to the conclusion that potassium alone is not as effective in producing results as potassium with associated minerals, some of which must activate the potassium.

"One reason for the versatility of apple cider vinegar as a remedy in Vermont folk medicine is that it associates minerals with potassium. These are phosphorus, chlorine, sodium, magnesium, calcium, sulfur, iron, fluorine, silicon and trace minerals."

And the second reason vinegar makes potassium so effective is that it presents the mineral in an acid medium, "and nature always combines potassium with an acid. I'd have to guess potassium needs an acid medium to work," Blodgett said.

Proper Growth

"Drink your vinegar and you'll grow up big and strong," is probably not something you heard in your house when you were a child, but it would have been absolutely true had your mother said it.

Potassium's main function is to promote cell, tissue and organism growth. This also means that potassium is necessary to replace worn-out tissue and dead cells. Basically, *it sustains life.* Slow growth in a child — or a failure to grow — could well be a sign of potassium deficiency, and so are signs of premature aging such as loss of hair, tooth decay, or fingernails that are either brittle and tear, or soft and bend. That means that both young and old alike need plenty of potassium.

"Potassium requirements are at a maximum when they are being used in infancy to build body tissues. But the requirements continue throughout life and there is no substitute for potassium," Jarvis writes.

And there is no better source of potassium than vinegar — particularly that apple cider vinegar.

Strong Circulation

As long as you can keep your circulation system free from obstructions, and keep your blood flowing freely, you dramatically reduce your risk of suffering a heart attack. The slow accumulation of fat and plaque deposits inside the blood vessels eventually chokes off the blood supply, and hardens veins and arteries that need to be strong yet supple.

The major culprit for this process is our usually out-of-balance diet.

But apple cider vinegar can help.

"...There is very little doubt that one of the functions of potassium is to keep the tissue soft and pliable," Jarvis notes. "Potassium is to the soft tissues what calcium is to the hard tissues (bones) of the body. There is little doubt that potassium slows up the hardening processes that menace the whole blood vessel system."

One of the side benefits tied to improved circulation is clearer thinking. Mental activity is more effective because more oxygen reaches the brain. One of potassium's many benefits is that it promotes oxygenation of the blood.

Infection Fighter

Vinegar can help you fight off infections by keeping fluids where they belong: In your body cells, and not in bacteria.

Here's the way that works. Bacteria need moisture to thrive. They pull fluids out of your body's cells for their own purposes. If they multiply and your resistance is down, the process can go unchecked and you can become very sick. The ultimate end result of this process is death, naturally, but there are fortunately a number of medicines available today to prevent that.

The way to defeat bacterial infections, then, is to keep moisture in the cells and not the germs get to it.

According to Dr. Jarvis: "If there is enough potassium in each body cell, it will draw moisture from the bacteria, instead of the bacteria taking moisture from the body cells ...It is by taking care to eat foods which are a source of potassium, such as fruit, berries, edible leaves, edible roots and honey, and by the use of apple cider vinegar that the body cells are provided with the moisture-attracting potassium needed to win the contest with bacteria."

35

In addition, Dr. Blodgett explained to me that many of the medicines used to combat bacterial illnesses work on the same principle: by depriving bacteria of moisture and thus keeping fluids inside the cells.

Though the simple language of Dr. Jarvis may sound somewhat old-fashioned compared to the convoluted medical and scientific terminology we have become accustomed to today, from more than thirty years ago it still expresses an important modern truth. And it is refreshing to think that in this age of nuclear medicine and high-tech tests that can cost as much as $1,500 that the horse-sense of a country doctor may be just as helpful as many of the complex medical procedures that are available today.

Healthy Digestion

Good digestion means health. Two teaspoonfuls of apple cider vinegar to a glass of water at each meal is helpful in maintaining the health of your digestive tract, and in turn, the all-around health of your body.

Apple cider vinegar destroys micro-organisms, including bacteria, fungi, viruses and others, and prevents poisons from reaching the rest of your system.

This effect is so potent that it can even protect you from food poisoning, if you accidentally eat some fish, meat or other food that has spoiled slightly. Of course, it is always better to eat good, fresh food and avoid the problem in the first place. But it is helpful to know that you can avoid discomfort if you are accidentally sidelined.

This is especially useful information for the summer picnic season, which is also prime time for food poisoning. Unsuspecting vacationers can end a day of swimming, tennis and horseshoes writhing in agony from diarrhea and the rest of these wickedly upsetting digestive crises.

During the warm months, people who like to enjoy the outdoors also bring along lots of foods — which they leave standing unrefrigerated, thus giving bacteria a wonderful opportunity to firmly take charge. The apple cider vinegar treatment can make the difference between normal digestion and illness.

And in cases of inadvertent consumption of contaminated food, a teaspoon of apple cider vinegar added to a glass of water can treat the illness when it's usually too late — when symptoms are already present. "When there is food poisoning with vomiting, if you should attempt to drink a whole glass at once, the stomach will not accept it. But a small amount every few minutes can be kept down.

"And ordinary drinking glass will hold about fifty teaspoonsful, and teaspoonful doses will require about four hours. When the contents of the first glass have been taken, another should be prepared in the same way and the dose increased to two or more teaspoonsful every five minutes. This will add another two hours of treatment. A third glassful should be prepared and taken one small swallow every fifteen minutes," recommends Jarvis.

If you wake up with nausea and vomiting or other symptoms of digestive upsets, he advises following the apple cider vinegar and water treatment throughout the day. By suppertime, you should be able to eat something light and easily digestible. Be sure to take extra vinegar and water five times a day or more for the next three days.

Kidney And Bladder

Apple cider vinegar keeps these organs doing their vital work of eliminating waste from the body.

It combats inflammation of the kidneys, which can lead to a backup of toxins, and eventually to blood poisoning.

The acid nature of vinegar makes the environment in the urinary tract inhospitable to germs. Two teaspoons of vinegar in water will even quiet a potentially dangerous condition called pyelitis, in which pus cells originating in the bladder are present in the urine.

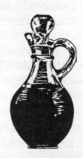

6 Vanishing Fat and Other Good News

Everybody's looking for the magic bullet that will allow them to eat steak subs and french fries, with ice cream for dessert and still stay skinny.

Well, I'm afraid that I do have to let you know that apple cider vinegar is not such a magic bullet, so don't hold your breath.

But it can do something very important for you in your determination to get slim — or stay slim. Apple cider vinegar can help kick that metabolism of your into a higher gear. And that means that your body is more likely to burn fat, than to store it as unsightly flab. So there is a lot of good news for you here, and, again, you have the potassium content to give thanks to, because it is potassium that promotes the proper chemical reactions in your body. And the acid nature of the vinegar makes certain that the conditions your body requires for fat burning are just right.

Do I hear you say that you're not sure if you are overweight or not? Well, these days we have all kinds of help. We have digital scales, insurance company weight tables linked to height, and so on and so on. It's all around us. Dr. Jarvis looked at it in a rather more old fashioned, homespun fashion.

"If the waist measurement is greater than that of the chest, or the chin is inclined to be double, then it is generally safe to conclude that the normal physiology and biochemistry in the body are disturbed." Read: You're too fat if it takes more tape to measure around your waist or hips than your chest.

"When this happens Vermont folk medicine depends on apple cider vinegar to bring about a disappearance of fat."

The good news is that you don't have to make any frightening, major alterations in your daily diet. Just make sure, honestly, that you take care to avoid those foods that your experience has shown absolutely pack on the pounds around your waistline or your hips. For most people, sweets, chips, other snacks and burgers are likely to be the prime culprits. I know they are from my own experience. But don't ever let me hear you say that it is bread, potatoes or pasta that make you fat, because they really do not.

Fat is fattening, and starchy foods such as those simply do not contain any fat. Meats, whole milk and cheese, pastries, snacks and junk food are the prime sources of fat, and the principle. And so it is always the butter, sour cream or cheese that you add to starchy foods that actually put the weight. It definitely is not the bread, spaghetti or the potatoes.

The less than wonderful news is that vinegar cannot help you lose ten pounds in ten days. The actual weight loss will be gradual, and that is really good news because researchers have shown over and over that it is weight that is lost gradually that stays off.

"If a woman between five feet and five feet six inches tall weighing 210 pounds ...takes two teaspoonfuls of apple cider vinegar in a glass of water at each meal, she will weigh about 180 pounds at the end of two years. If a man has a paunch, he will lose the paunch in two years' time."

Slim Down

Since the vinegar will be helping you burn fat instead of store it, your daily activities will help you shed inches (and rolls) much more quickly than pounds.

"If a woman whose dress fits tightly will sip two teaspoonsful of apple cider vinegar in a glass of water at each meal she will find at the end of two months that she can take her dress in one inch at the waistline. At the end of two more months she will be able to take it in another inch, and by the end of the fifth month one more inch. At the end of one year of taking apple cider vinegar in this amount a woman who has taken a size 50 dress will be able to take a size 42, and one who has taken a size 20, to take a size 18. At the end of the same time a younger woman who has worn a size 16 will be able to take a size 14."

Dr. Blodgett called the weight loss plan completely simple and completely effective. It certainly sounds easy.

Chronic fatigue is like an alarm clock waking you from sound sleep: It alerts you that a dramatic change must take place quickly. This is a fancy way of saying fatigue is a warning sign of impending illness.

Sleep Deficit

A recent study at Cornell University showed that over 50 million Americans are suffering from sleep deficit and the resultant fatigue. Translation: They don't sleep enough. The solution, of course, is to get more sleep.

Most of us are yawning and dragging around with heavy eyelids most of the time because there is so much to do in this get-up-and-go society of ours. When Dr. Blodgett would see the circles under my eyes, he would point out to me that I should go to bed earlier. He would add that artificial lighting is a relatively new invention, and that in the days before Thomas Edison, people used to go to bed not long after sunset and wake with the sunrise. Obviously times have changed, and that is no longer possible or practical. But all of us could do with an hour more sleep a night.

But above all, you want to stay away from sedatives, sleeping pills, narcotics or alcohol to help you.

Once again, it's apple cider vinegar to the rescue.

"To cope with chronic fatigue," Jarvis reports, "Vermont folk medicine knows no better treatment than this: add three teaspoonsful of apple cider vinegar to a cup of honey, placing the mixture in a wide-mouthed bottle or jar that will admit a teaspoon, and keep the jar in the bedroom. Take two teaspoonsful of the mixture when preparing for bed."

And so to Sleep

He says this should put you to sleep within a half-hour. If you're still staring at the ceiling, take two more teaspoonsful (it tastes good) and another at any time you wake up and feel unable to fall back asleep.

"This is far superior to the usual 'lullaby pills' because it is a treatment based on Nature's own infallible knowledge of bodily requirements; being harmless, it can be taken indefinitely. The honey may be taken by itself to produce sleep, but Vermont folk medicine teaches that the combining of it with the apple cider vinegar is more effective."

Another way to overcome fatigue is to use apple cider vinegar in your bath. Add a half pint to a tub full of bath water and immerse yourself in it for fifteen minutes. The skin will absorb some of the vinegar, and potassium along with it, and pep you up. One note: Use the vinegar in the bath water instead of soap. It will clean your skin quite effectively. Yet another way to perk yourself up is to add several ounces to a sinkful of water and to splash it on your shoulders, arms, in your armpits, on your chest, stomach, neck and face. Don't dry it with a towel, but let it soak in. You will find it quite refreshing.

Migraines, Tension..

For migraines, stress or tension headaches — or just about any type — apple cider vinegar is worth a try.

Many naturopath physicians believe that most headaches have a single cause: too much alkaline in the system. When the body chemistry is changed back to a natural acidity, headaches usually disappear or become mild and manageable.

Dr. Jarvis writes that you can restore that level of natural acidity by taking apple cider vinegar in water in the morning and evening and at every meal. If your headaches are bad, try doubling the amount of vinegar at first. He also recommends two teaspoonsful of honey at each meal to prevent a headache. "If the headache has appeared, however, take a tablespoon of honey at once. Since it requires no process of digestion and will quickly be in the blood stream, the headache will often begin to lessen by the end of a half hour. If not, another teaspoonful of honey should be taken."

A vinegar vapor is also effective in relieving migraines. Put equal parts apple cider vinegar and water in a pan on the stove, and bring it to a slow boil. Lean your head over, and inhale as the fumes begin to rise from the basin. "Inhale them for 75 breaths. Generally you will find that the headache stops for about a half hour. If it starts again it will be about 50 percent less severe. The use of headache tablets can be stopped if the apple cider vinegar fumes method is employed."

Blood Pressure

Modern research bears out the folklore. A diet high in protein — because most of our protein comes from meat, it's generally also high in fat — and low in carbohydrates is a major contributor to elevated blood pressure. Every major health organization in the country agrees with that assessment, recommending a low-fat, high-fiber diet (carbohydrates are the best sources of fiber) to combat the condition. This step will also prevent the likelihood of heart attacks and strokes that result from hypertension.

A high-protein/high-fat diet turns the blood alkaline, which thickens it. That is one of the primary contributing factors to high blood pressure. Apple cider vinegar converts the blood to acidity, thins it, lowers the blood pressure and makes circulation less of a strain.

Here is Jarvis's plan to lower high blood pressure:

1. Increase the daily intake of acid in organic form, either as apple cider vinegar, apples, grapes, cranberries or their juices.

2. Change to a more balanced diet. Ask the American Heart Association, the American Cancer Society or a local dietitian for guidelines to a heart-healthy diet that's low in fat and high in fiber. It will automatically give you an advantage in the war on high blood pressure.

3. Change from wheat products (breads, muffins, cereals) to corn, oats, rye or rice. They will assist the shift from alkalinity to acidity within you and reduce strain on your kidneys — kidney damage and eventual failure is an often-overlooked complication of high blood pressure.

4. Give up salt and salty foods. This will reverse the blood's tendency to retain so much fluid — a prime hypertension cause .

Sore Throats

An apple cider vinegar gargle brings marked relief to sore throats. Use one teaspoonful to a glass of water and gargle with a mouthful of the solution every hour. Then swallow the solution, so it reaches the lower parts of the throat you can't touch by gargling. Repeat with a second mouthful. As pain lessens, increase intervals between gargling to every two hours.

The gargling kills strep germs, Jarvis reports. "Much to my surprise I learned that this treatment could cure a streptococcic sore throat in 24 hours. As a rule the patient became free of symptoms even before the Vermont state laboratory confirmed that the culture showed the presence of streptococci."

By the way, the apple cider vinegar treatment can also eliminate uncomfortable and embarrassing post-nasal drip. This is caused by a production of excess mucus, which seeps out of the sinus cavities into the throat. It seems like a mere annoyance, but it is a perfect breeding ground for bacteria and other germs. If you suffer from this seemingly minor condition, it places you at more or less constant risk of a sore throat and upper respiratory infection.

Signs of a Potassium Deficiency

1. Loss of mental alertness; difficulty with decision making; lapses in memory

2. More frequent episodes of mental and muscle fatigue; loss of stamina and easy tiring

3. Sensitivity to cold and a propensity to cold hands and feet

4. Calluses on the bottom of the feet and growing corns

5. Constipation troubles

6. Susceptibility to sickness; frequent colds

7. Temporary losses of appetite with bouts of nausea and vomiting

8. Slow healing of cuts and bruises

9. Frequent and bothersome itches

10. Bothersome tooth decay

11. Pimples

12. Twitching of the eyelids or the corners of the mouth

13. Muscle cramps, especially in the legs, most often at night

14. Difficulty relaxing

15. Difficulty sleeping

16. Soreness in the joints; other symptoms of arthritis

If you detect more than five of these signs, you could be suffering from a potassium deficiency. While it may be advisable to see a physician, remember that as you grow older you need more potassium. Since this mineral is non-toxic, it's a good idea to increase your intake of it whether you see a doctor or not.

Increasing Potassium Intake

1. Shake paprika on your food once or twice a day — it's a rich source of potassium

2. Drink a glass of grape juice twice a day

3. Alternatives are a glass of apple or cranberry juice twice a day

4. Eat a large banana every day

5. Turn to grapefruits and other citrus as often as they're in season

6. Eat two large potatoes each day (baked, boiled or cooked in some other way that does not laden them with fat)

7. Eat two or three raw carrots a day

8. Add tomatoes to your salad and tomato sauce to your pasta

9. Eat at least two salads a day. Go heavy on the leafy greens, especially spinach, watercress, escarole, romaine lettuce and other dark leafy greens

10. When cantalope is in season, make it a regular treat

11. Snack on sunflower seeds

Vitamin Bible

Dr. Earl Mindell, author of *The Vitamin Bible* (Warner, $4.95) says that alcohol, coffee, sugar and diuretics are the enemies of potassium. If you drink large amounts of coffee, you may ironically find yourself frequently the victim of fatigue. That is the direct result of potassium depletion. The solution is to increase potassium consumption at the same time reducing the amount of coffee you consume every day.

Arthritis

Apple cider vinegar, taken on a daily basis, can bring you arthritis relief by helping to dissolve calcium deposits in joints and whisking them away for excretion.

As the blood becomes alkaline and thick, the solid particles in it precipitate out, and drop where they may in the body. For example, fat and cholesterol particles, blood clots, calcium and other materials, filter out of the bloodstream to form hard and deadly atherosclerotic plaque on the inside walls of the arteries. In the same way, calcium may form deposits inside joints, making movement difficult and painful, and causing inflammation.

Jarvis, quoting folk healers in his native New England and backing them up from his own research, believes that by taking apple cider vinegar and water every day, you lower your blood's natural alkalinity, bringing it closer to an acid state. This may dissolve calcium deposits and ease arthritis discomfort.

Anyone suffering from the excruciating pain of any one of the many forms that arthritis takes, may well find relief in following his advice.

Best of All, It's "Green"

The long list of chemicals and additives you will find in most detergents and cleaners today may well be hazardous to your health. They are certainly dangerous to any child who wanders into a cupboard filled with drain cleaner, spot remover or floor wax — and drinks some or splashes some in the eyes. And once you throw the dregs down the drain or toss the packaging in the garbage (which means years, possibly centuries, in a landfill), these chemicals and materials harm the earth.

Luckily, there are environmentally safe products for housework and they are just as effective as anything you can buy — in most cases a lot cheaper. In fact, you probably have many of them in your kitchen already: baking soda, lemon juice, vegetable oil, borax and old-fashioned hot water.

At the head of the list, put vinegar. Just look at the many ways it can be used:

Air freshening: commercial air fresheners work by deadening nerves in your nose to diminish your sense of smell, not the odors. Set two to four tablespoons of vinegar in open dishes instead.

Dishwashing liquids: the number one cause of child poisoning among household products. And they're mostly made of non-biodegradable detergents, with lots of chemical additives. Use liquid or powdered soap such as Ivory instead, adding two to three teaspoons of vinegar for heavy cleaning power.

Drain cleaners: usually containing lye, hydrochloric and sulfuric acids, they can disfigure you. Once a week, plug the overflow drain with a wet rag, pour a quarter cup baking soda down the drain and follow with one-half cup of vinegar. Close the drain until the fizzing stops. Flush with one gallon of boiling water.

Floor cleaners: one half cup of vinegar (white, preferably) mixed in a half gallon of warm water cuts through dull, greasy film on no-wax linoleum.

Furniture polish: many wood polishes contain phenol, which caused cancer during laboratory tests on rats. So mix vegetable oil (or lemon oil) and vinegar in equal parts and apply as a thin coat. Rub in well.

Glass cleaner: commercial products contain ammonia, which is a poison. Try this instead: use alcohol first to clean off the residue of other cleaners, then clean glass with a mixture of white vinegar and warm water in equal proportions.

Metal polishes: most contain phosphoric and sulfuric acids and pollute the indoor air. For aluminum, soak overnight in a mixture of vinegar and water, then rub. For brass, mix equal parts of salt and flour with a little vinegar, then rub. For chrome, rub with undiluted vinegar. For copper, rub with a paste of vinegar, salt and flour, or hot vinegar and salt.

Mold and mildew: to avoid the harmful pesticides likely to be ingredients in commercial products designed to tackle these growths, make a concentrated solution of borax or vinegar and water to clean the affected areas. When you're sure it's mildew, try a mixture of vinegar and salt first.

Toilet cleaners: the blueing agent you buy in your local supermarket or corner store contains chlorine and hydrochloric acid which can burn your eyes and burn holes in your skin. Use soap and borax to remove stubborn rings, and white vinegar to remove lime buildup. Another option is to sprinkle baking soda into the bowl, drizzle with vinegar and scour with a toilet brush.

7 Making Vinegar at Home

Vinegar: 1. a sour liquid used as a condiment or preservative that is obtained by acetic fermentation of dilute alcoholic liquids (as fermented cider, malt beer, or wine) or of dilute distilled alcohol and is often seasoned, esp. with herbs 2. disagreeableness of speech, disposition or attitude 3. a pharmaceutical solution of the active principles of drugs in dilute acetic acid usu., prepared by maceration

Webster's Dictionary

You can quite easily make your own apple cider vinegar — or blackberry vinegar — and you can add tasty herbs to commercially prepared vinegars that you can buy in any supermarket.

In her superb book *Herbal Medicine*, Dr. Dian Dincin Buchman, Ph.D., of the State University of New York at Purchase and at the College of New Rochelle, who is one of the most noted writers and lecturers on the benefits of natural medicine in the world, enthuses about the benefits of vinegars.

She recommends this invigorating drink which relieves fatigue and also helps to dissolve arthritic and gouty deposits: Combine a tablespoon of uncooked honey and a tablespoon of a good apple cider vinegar. Add this mixture to a glass of water. You may use a little less honey if you are making a pitcherful. This excellent drink is good for small children (although not for newborn infants) and

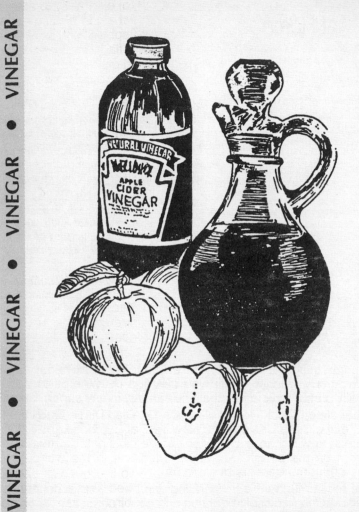

this ancient combination of sweet and sour plus water normalizes the body.

She writes: "Apple cider vinegar is useful externally to alleviate pain and help reduce sprains. I use at least a cup at a time in the bath to alleviate muscle soreness. I also splash it directly on my shoulders, arms, chest, and torso to restore flagging energy. I don't really know why apple cider vinegar patted on the body or placed in the bathwater will overcome body fatigue, but it does.

"Diluted apple cider vinegar may be used in small amounts to help reduce fever and may also be splashed or sponged on the patient to reduce the temperature. Carefully sponge the body in sections and friction dry, and do not allow the rest of the body to be in a draft."

Herb vinegars are also excellent when used to cleanse sick-rooms and wash the patient during any bacterial illness or during an epidemic of any kind.

Doing it Yourself

You will need a wide-mouthed jar or crock, a cover for the crock, and the peelings, cores, and bruised apples left after making apple sauce or apple pie, writes Dr. Buchman. Place the leftover pieces of apple in the crock, and cover with cold water. Place the top on the crock, and store it in a warm place. Occasionally lift the cover and add whatever additional peels, cores, and apple pieces you can. Strain off the froth as you go along. When the vinegar smells and tastes right, strain out the apple pieces. Pour the vinegar into sterilized bottles, and cork for further use.

Aeration is the answer to souring a vinegar. If you wish to quicken the fermentation process, add a small amount of live yeast in a brown paper bag to your crock or keg.

To aerate as farmers once did, keep two barrels with spigots. In one barrel, make the vinegar as described above. In the second barrel, keep matchstick-thin sticks of birch or beech boards. After a few days, open the faucet and allow the cider to dribble through the birch or beech boards. As soon as the second barrel fills up, pour the vinegar into the first barrel again. This process may be repeated several times.

Some Vinegars

Here are some of Dr. Buchman's favorite vinegar recipes that you can try:

Blackberry Vinegar

4 lbs fresh blackberries
Enough malt vinegar to cover blackberries
1 lb sugar for every pint of extracted blackberry juice*

*Sugar can be replaced with glycerine. See the recipe for Blackberry Glycerite.

Wash the blackberries in cold running water. Place in a glass, earthenware, or ceramic pot. Cover with malt vinegar for three days. Stir once a day. Strain through a sieve, and drain thoroughly by placing a plate on top and putting a weight on the plate. Let it drip all day. Measure the juice, and allow one pound of sugar per pint of juice (for external use, glycerine is preferred—see next recipe). Simmer in another glass, ceramic, or earthenware pot for five minutes. Collect and discard the top scum. Cool, bottle, cork, and label.

Dr. Buchman reports that this vinegar is excellent for fevers, arthritis, and gout. The dosage here is one tablespoon dissolved in a large cup of distilled water. Use three times a day. This preparation will somewhat ease the pain, and is said to eventually help dissolve arthritic deposits. This vinegar is also said to be good for anemia and may be used with advantage by many heart patients.

Blackberry Glycerite

The recipe for this is almost the same as that for blackberry vinegar, but glycerine is used instead of the sugar. For every pint of the extracted juice, use 8 ounces of glycerine (½ pint). Simmer the blackberry vinegar and glycerine together for five minutes. Skim. Cool and place in a sterilized, labeled bottle. Store in a cool place.

This glycerite of blackberry can be used in the same way as the vinegar. For painful joints, heat this preparation in small quantities, dip in a folded cloth. Several times a day apply hot cloths to painful joints.

Vinegar of the Four Thieves

This is one of the most interesting legends in the fascinating history of herbalism, reports Dr. Buchman. She says that the recipe may have been actually devised by an apothecary, Richard Forthave, and that the success and usefulness of the remedy created its own myth. This recipe has been in use for centuries, but the legend has it that it was discovered during a devastating bubonic plague.

Four thieves who had safely ransacked empty plague-ridden houses were caught by policemen and brought before the French judges in Marseilles. The judges wondered aloud how these thieves had resisted the plague, especially since they were in and out of plague-infested homes.

"We drink and wash with this vinegar preparation every few hours," they answered.

In return for giving the recipe, the thieves were given their freedom.

There are several *Four Thieves vinegars*. Dr. Buchman extracted the simplest recipe from the notebook of a Virginia housewife. She combined a handful of each of the antidisease herbs and steeped them in apple cider vinegar. After the initial two-week steeping (a vinegar tincture), she added garlic buds.

This aromatic and antibacterial vinegar is an excellent wash for floors, walls, sinks, bedsteads, pots, and pans, in sickrooms, bathrooms, and kitchens. It will offset a damp-weather smell in a house and be a helpful floor and wall wash in a room overcrowded with people.

Externally, this vinegar may be used in small proportions in a bath or diluted for body wash. Ordinary apple cider vinegars may be used in an undiluted state if desired, but some of the herbs in this recipe are too strong for the skin, and the vinegar must be diluted.

Internally, the dose is a teaspoon at a time in water — no more than one tablespoon an hour (three teaspoons equals one tablespoon). This acts as a preventive during an epidemic.

Vinegar of the Four Thieves

2 qts apple cider vinegar
2 tbs lavender
2 tbs rosemary
2 tbs sage
2 tbs wormwood
2 tbs rue
2 tbs mint
2 tbs garlic buds

Combine the dried herbs (except the garlic), and steep in the vinegar in the sun for two weeks. Strain and rebottle. Label. Add several cloves of garlic. Close lid. When garlic has steeped for several days, strain out. Melt paraffin wax around the lid to preserve the contents, or add 4 ounces of glycerine for preservation.

Note dosage above.

Modern Anti-Epidemic Vinegar

1 quart apple cider vinegar
1 lb garlic buds for 8 oz juice
8 oz comfrey root
4 oz oak bark
4 oz marshmallow root
4 oz mullein flowers
4 oz rosemary flowers
4 oz lavender flowers
4 oz wormwood
4 oz black walnut leaves
12 oz glycerine

Make separate teas of each of the herbs. First soak each ounce of herb in clean spring water. After about half a day, simmer each herb separately for ten minutes. Steep for a half hour. Strain out, simmer again, and reduce each herb so that it is concentrated. Press garlic buds into 8 ounces of concentrated juice. Add 12 ounces of glycerine to preserve it. Place in a large bottle. Label. Close. You may want to add paraffin for additional preservation power.

Dosage: 1-3 tsp during epidemics, or 1 tsp per hour if someone in the family is ill with a communicable disease. Dilute with water if too strong to the taste, or add to hot herbal tea.

Herb Vinegars for Face, Bath, or Salad

Here are four more excellent herb vinegar recipes. You can use them as a refreshing, aromatic addition to bath water, or as in invigorating facial splash. They also make delightful dressings for salads.

1 qt apple cider vinegar
4 tbs dried herbs (or 2 tbs fresh herbs)

Place vinegar in a ceramic or glass pot. Bring to a brief boil. Turn off heat. Add herbs. Pour into vinegar jar. Use leftover vinegar for body wash or addition to bath.

● ● ●

1 qt apple cider vinegar
1 handful fresh mint or tarragon (or 3 tbs dried mint)

Wash mint, bruise leaves well, and pack into jar. Cover tightly, and let stand two weeks. Strain out the herbs. (If dried mint is used, first simmer the vinegar, bring to a boil, and then pour over the mint.)

● ● ●

½ pint apple cider vinegar
1 oz rose petals
½ pint rosewater
½ pint vinegar (apple cider or white)
1 oz several different kinds of aromatic flowers (examples: lavender, sweet violet, rosemary)

Mix and steep for two weeks.

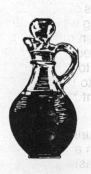

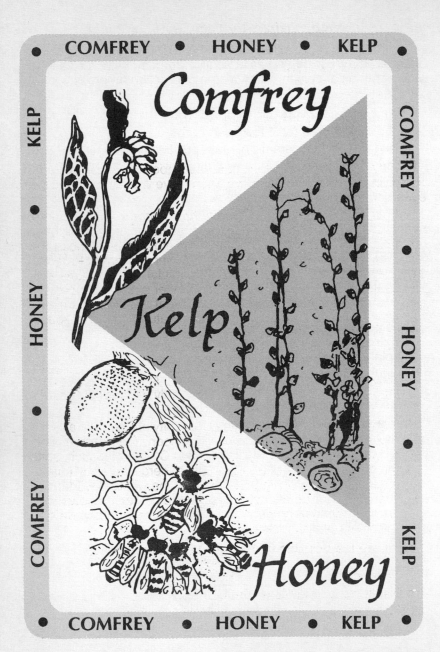

8 Honey, Kelp and Comfrey

Always remember: Nature has been good to us, amply supplying us with everything we need, if we would only open our eyes and use our heads.

With that in mind, let's look at the three natural wonders in the chapter title. They are, in turn, a bee's nectar, a seaweed and an aromatic herb. When you integrate them into a well-balanced diet they can counteract stress, soothe raw nerves, promote restful sleep, kill bacteria and other germs, stimulate the immune system, increase resistance to cancer and other modern ills, prevent heart disease, and disinfect wounds. And that doesn't include their well-known talent for flavoring beverages, natural desserts, soups, stews, and other dishes.

Honey

Cynics say honey's nothing but a simple sugar, no better than the white powder in your sugar bowl and only a fool would believe differently.

But what about researchers at the University of Colorado at Boulder, the University of Wisconsin at Madison, Georgetown University Medical Center, in Washington, D.C., the Massachusetts Institute of Technology (M.I.T.), and Heidelberg University (one of the oldest institutions of higher learning in the western world) and elsewhere? Scientists at each one of those centers have verified at least one healthful property of honey. It's hard to believe that these scholars are all fools!

Here are the possible therapeutic benefits of honey:

- Kills bacteria
- Disinfects wounds and sores
- Eases the perception of pain

- Alleviates asthma
- Soothes sore throats
- Calms the nerves
- Induces sleep
- Relieves diarrhea

Dr. Jarvis says honey is an everyday type of health tonic and recommends it for coughs, sore throats, muscle cramps, burns, stuffy noses, sinusitis, hay fever and other allergies, insomnia and bed-wetting in children.

British researchers have proven that applying honey directly to open wounds keeps them sterile and prevents infections, gangrene and other complications as well as any medication known, if not better. In fact, honey can often eliminate the need for conventional (and costly) antibiotics.

Prominent surgeons writing in the prestigious medical journal *The Lancet* say that honey-covered wounds heal faster and support less bacterial colonization than wounds treated with ordinary antibiotics. Test tube experiments showed honey kills a wide range of infectious micro-organisms.

Why? You might ask. We'll let Dr. Jarvis explain. "It's no mere theory but has been proven that bacteria cannot live in the presence of honey for the reason that honey is an excellent source of potassium." Potassium again.

Subsequent research has suggested that honey may have more going for it than just potassium. Chemical analysis at the University of Wisconsin showed copper, iron and manganese to be present in honey in respectable amounts. Iron, especially, is very important for sustaining the red coloring matter in blood called hemoglobin, which has the task of transporting oxygen to all tissues in the body.

These minerals are present in relatively slight quantities, but it is widely accepted that numerous minerals are needed by the human body in very small amounts to keep the body in mineral balance.

Honey is also rich in vitamin C, riboflavin, nicotinic acid and other B vitamins, which accounts for honey's widely reported abilities to calm down highly-strung people and to promote a good night's sleep. "A tablespoon of honey at the evening meal makes you look forward to bedtime," writes Jarvis.

Honey is also predigested, reducing the amount of work your stomach has to do so that the body can use it. While this is of relatively little importance to healthy individuals, it can mean a great deal to people with impaired digestion.

Here are the advantages of honey over other simple sugars:

- It is non-irritating to the lining of the digestive tract

- It is easily and rapidly assimilated

- It quickly answers the demand for energy

- It helps athletes, laborers and anyone else who expends large amounts of energy to recuperate rapidly from exertion

- It places the least strain on the kidneys of all sugars

- It has a natural and gentle laxative effect

- It has sedative value, quieting the body

- It is easily obtainable and widely available

- It is inexpensive

So, doctors might like you to believe honey is no different than white sugar, but don't you believe them.

"Honey will, by several effects, render old age less difficult to live," Dr. Jarvis writes. "I am saddened when people tell me that they don't eat honey because it costs more than white sugar. I try to make them see that health is not to be had for the asking. Good health is earned. In the long run you must pay either the grocer or the drug store. When you become sick, you find you must spend the money you saved on food to purchase drugs to bring back your health. By purchasing the right kind of food, such as honey represents, you can constructively cut some corners."

Now, how's that for good old-fashioned, common sense?

Honey in Infant Formula

While nothing compares to mother's milk, honey can make infant formula come closer. If, for whatever reason, a mother is unable to nurse, fortifying the infant's food with honey will achieve positive results.

Jarvis recommends one to two teaspoonsful of honey in eight ounces of feeding mixture. "Infants fed on honey rarely have colic; the rapid absorption of honey prevents fermentation from taking place."

He believes the potassium it supplies is vital for the rapid growth of the baby's body. At the same time, honey is palatable, calming and full of minerals. Because of the nature of its sugars, honey provides both a quick energy release and a slow energy release which maintains the baby's blood glucose level, avoiding the swings and crashes one would see with processed sugar.

Studies at the Universities of Minnesota and Chicago confirmed these observations, and doctors at these research centers say honey ought to be more widely used in infant feeding.

Honey And Bed-Wetting

Bed-wetting is quite normal in the first three years of life, but when it continues beyond that age, it needs some attention.

Obviously, physical training in the ways of bladder control are necessary for prevention. But honey, it may surprise you, is an effective, natural, inexpensive, and tasty treatment your child will love, Jarvis says.

"At bedtime give the child a teaspoonful of honey. It will act in two ways. First, it will act as a sedative to the nervous system. Second...it will attract and hold fluid during the hours of sleeping." Try it every night at first until you notice results. Then observe what conditions are likely to produce an episode of bed-wetting. High excitement and stimulation plus lots of liquid intake are prime suspects. Hold honey in reserve for those occasions, and use it as a preventive treatment.

Cough Remedy

Boil one lemon slowly for 10 minutes. Cut in two and extract the juice with a lemon squeezer (the softened rind and pulp will yield a larger quantity of juice than a lemon straight out of the refrigerator). Pour the juice into a glass or jar and add enough honey so the mixture thickens (if you can obtain glycerin at a pharmacy, add two tablespoonsful). If you have no lemons, use apple cider vinegar. Take a teaspoonful when you wake up, in the middle of the morning, with the midday meal, in the midafternoon, after supper and at bedtime. It does not upset the stomach, is safe for children as well as effective for adults, and it works.

Muscle Cramps

At times we may be plagued by an annoying twitching of the eyelids or at the corner of the mouth. It can soon be made to disappear by the taking of two teaspoonsful of honey at each meal. As a rule, it will disappear within a week's time.

Honey For Burns

Apply it directly to steam burns, and burns from open flames or hot objects. It relieves the stinging and smarting, stops the formation of blisters, prevents infection, produces rapid healing and keeps scarring to a minimum.

Honey is a sugar, and if you use too much it can contribute to weight gain. Be moderate in the amounts you consume.

For those of you thinking that honey sounds so old-fashioned, stop for a minute and think of all the modern remedies for burns, blisters, bed-wetting, coughs, cuts, colds, hay-fever and the like. How well do they work? Most doctors will admit not that well. Even when they do work, just read the list of contraindications (risks and hazards) and you'll see that sometimes the treatment may be worse than the cure.

Honey is food. And a natural wonder. And if all the analysis leaves you cold and the fancy explanations don't clear up the mystery of honey or convince you it's useful, take comfort in the words of Dr. Blodgett, "Who cares why it works? It just does. Honey's got something in it that's clearly very good for you."

And that about sums it up.

Kelp

Kelp is an old-time word for seaweed. It's powerful stuff.

Modern science confirms that seaweed is an all-around wonder, nutritionally, medically and pharmaceutically. Here are a few of its astounding health benefits:

- Kills bacteria
- Smothers cancer
- Fortifies the immune system
- Heals ulcers

- Lowers cholesterol levels
- Reduces blood pressure
- Prevents strokes
- Thins the blood

The reason for this expansive talent is simple: Almost every chemical known on earth dissolves in the oceans. This means that plant and animal life growing in the sea is not deficient in any of the elements necessary to support life. In this day and age, the one drawback to the ocean acting as a depository for all the chemicals on earth is that it collects pollution, toxic wastes and garbage as well as life-sustaining minerals, metals and elements. But most scientists still think the benefits of seafood (fish and kelp) far outweigh the drawbacks.

And folk medicine users have intuitively known for centuries what modern science is just now discovering: Kelp is a health treasure.

An Illustrious History

Throughout history, people have had tremendous luck and great results using kelp to treat constipation, bronchitis, emphysema, asthma, indigestion, ulcers, colitis, gallstones, obesity, and disorders of the genito-urinary and reproductive systems, both male and female, according to Dr. Varro Tyler, Dean of the School of Pharmacy, Nursing and Health Sciences, at Purdue University, in Lafayette, Indiana.

The claims for kelp also extend to being able to clean the bloodstream, strengthen disease resistance, quell arthritis and rheumatism discomfort, soothe and calm frayed nerves, counteract stress, and treat skin diseases, burns and insect bites, he adds.

Studies in the past two decades have clearly shown that many of these claims have a firm basis in fact. Kelp contains chemicals that can prevent and treat several types of cancer, curb high cholesterol and high blood pressure (the two prime culprits of heart disease), thin the blood, short-circuit ulcers, kill germs and cure constipation (as a plant it is very high in fiber).

Why? No one explains it better than Dr. Jarvis: "When seafood, either plant or animal, is eaten, these minerals are reabsorbed and perform their marvelous chemical functions of regulation and correction. The numerous elements coming from the sea, one of the most important of which is iodine, furnish the final essential link in the balanced diet.

He explains that the most essential mineral elements of body composition, in the order of their apparent importance, are iodine, copper, calcium, phosphorus, manganese, sodium, potassium, magnesium, chlorine and sulfur. All of these except iodine, which is a native of the sea, have their source in the soil. We would naturally suppose that when we eat products of the soil we should secure an ample supply of them. That is, no doubt, what Nature intended.

But Nature did not foresee that man would remove the trees and other growth, allowing the rains to erode the soil. This leaches out the essential minerals and, by means of our creeks and rivers, carries them down to the sea. The result is mineral-starved soil, which in turn produces food deficient in minerals. Stresses Jarvis: "The obvious result is that humans, who depend upon these mineral-starved foods for our supply of minerals, are literally starving in the midst of plenty."

The long and short of this is that when somebody tells you vitamin and mineral supplements are unnecessary — that a "balanced diet" supplies everything you need, they are wrong. That would be true if the land and soil were still at full strength, but we have weakened it. The soil in turn has yielded flimsy food, which is slowly wilting our vitality when we rely on it.

Kelp and Cancer

The Japanese eat vast quantities of seaweed. Epidemiologists have noted that Japanese women have a mere fraction of the breast cancers American women develop; and Japanese women who do fall prey to breast cancer live longer than American or British women with the disease. The scientists could not help wondering if there were a connection between high seaweed consumption and breast cancer protection.

Dr. Jane Teas of the Harvard School of Public Health checked out this theory. Her animal experiments showed that the brown seaweed *Laminaria* conferred protection against known cancer-causing chemicals.

The American Health Foundation, in Valhalla, New York, duplicated the findings, with even better results.

A Japanese study from 1974 showed that not only could kelp prevent the development of breast cancer, but that it could also treat tumors that had already begun growing. Kelp slowed the progression of breast malignancies in 95 percent of test animals. Sixty-six percent of them went into complete remission.

Dr. Teas speculates that the chemical called *fucoidan* in seaweed may play a large role in the anti-cancer capacity of kelp, but she notes that seaweeds also have potent antibiotic properties. That means seaweed may have promise in preventing or treating colon cancer, too.

A study at the University of Hawaii School of Medicine, in Honolulu, showed that a health food popular in Japan, a dried version of the seaweed, wakame, helped cure and prevent lung cancer when injected into laboratory animals. Researchers there found evidence that active ingredients in the seaweed activate the immune system.

Scientists have isolated blood pressure lowering (hypotensive) chemicals, including histamine, in kelp. Seaweed appears to act as an antidote to excess sodium consumption and may well help prevent strokes.

Kelp tablets are available in many health food stores, as are packaged seaweeds for cooking purposes. A single kelp tablet per day will give you all the minerals you need.

Comfrey

Herbs were probably the first healing agents used by humans. And comfrey is an herbal ace. Some experts consider it one of the most powerful healing herbs. It is so potent that it is best for external applications, although it sometimes figures in recipes for healing teas.

Herbalists recommend comfrey for:

- Healing wounds

- Disinfecting cuts

- Reducing bruises

- Shrinking phlebitis and venous clots

- Smoothing facial wrinkles

- Soothing respiratory ailments

62 • Easing digestive ills

The name comfrey is derived from the Latin word *confervere* that means to heal or knit together. It has also been called bruisewort, knitbone and healing herb. Because of the miraculous healing powers attributed to its roots and leaves, is one of the most commonly used herbs in traditional European and American folk medicine.

Comfrey is a member of the borage family of plants. It is found in damp environments and is native to Europe, western Siberia and the British Isles. It grows to a height of three to four feet, has long, oval leaves covered with sticky hairs, clusters of bell-shaped flowers and a bulbous root. Amateur gatherers need to be careful. Comfrey can easily be confused with foxglove because of its similar appearance, a mistake which can be serious, or on occasion, even fatal.

Healing Ointments

Researchers report that comfrey ointment or poultices heal almost any kind of sore, bruise or scrape. It also works wonders on insect bites and burns. To make an ointment, mix the powdered comfrey into any soft-based salve such as petroleum jelly, lanolin, wax, butter or lard. A poultice is a dampened cloth topped with the herb, in this case comfrey, which is spread over the affected area. Sometimes, as with mustard plasters, you place the herb between two dampened sheets to prevent any falling onto bare skin, which can cause irritation.

For simple cuts soak comfrey leaves in hot water and apply directly to the cut. Leave them in place for one hour.

Dr. Shlomo Noy, MD, of Tel Aviv University, in Israel, recommends a strong comfrey ointment for phlebitis (a blood clot lodged in a leg vein, such as Richard Nixon suffered while President).

He recommends a comfrey decoction two or three times a day for emphysema, bronchitis, asthma and pleurisy. This clears sputum and facilitates breathing. A decoction is similar to an infusion or tea, except you boil the herbs slower and longer (ten to fifteen minutes) in a covered pot and let them steep for 10 minutes. This is necessary to release the chemical properties.

And as a treatment for wrinkling and a brisk and invigorating facial splash, he recommends applying comfrey lotion twice a day, in the morning and again at night.

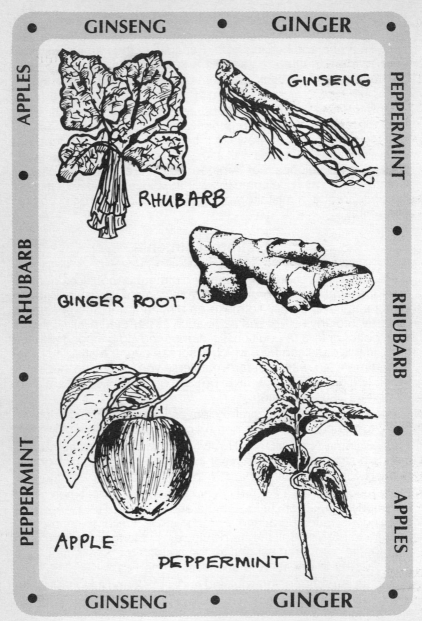

GINSENG

RHUBARB

GINGER ROOT

APPLE

PEPPERMINT

9 Try These Other Natural Wonders

An apple a day won't just keep the doctor away, it can also chase away the blues. A study at Michigan State University revealed that subjects who ate two apples a day had less tension, fewer headaches and less frequent emotional upsets, writes Ben Harris, author of *Home Remedies, Cures And Kitchen Tricks* (Gramercy Publishing Company, 1985). And an apple a day will also keep away the dentist. Apples help cleanse teeth of decay-causing carbohydrates, like sugar, and stimulate the gums and saliva flow.

A juice extracted from the roots and lower stems of asparagus is said to be an effective kidney remedy. To extract the juice, simply simmer two heaping tablespoonsful of chopped asparagus roots and lower stems in one quart of hot water for approximately 30 minutes, then strain. Drink a cupful every three to four hours.

Celery is another excellent vegetable for settling nerves, Harris points out in his no-nonsense book. Try the expressed juice of celery leaves and stalks in half cup doses, three to four times a day.

The oil from mashed cloves can be used for settling nerves of a different sort — in an aching tooth that has lost its filling!

Dates soaked in warm water until cool are said to be a naturally gentle laxative. Chew them well and don't forget to drink the water they were soaking in. A small dose, of five or six dates, in the morning and at night should be sufficient.

Looking for a first-rate facial? Soak overnight one tablespoonful of rolled oats in two tablespoonsful of buttermilk, then add the beaten white of one egg. Spread over the face and neck and let the mixture settle for 20 to 30 minutes. Remove with a soft washcloth and warm cool water, and repeat twice a day.

Papaya is a wonder fruit. Besides being highly nutritious, it gives immediate relief of indigestion and dyspepsia. It also cleans out the intestinal tract, and banishes bad breath.

Strawberries are excellent for the teeth. They prevent tartar build up, and dissolve tartar that has already taken hold. Halve the strawberry and rub it over the teeth. Allow the juice to stay on the teeth a minute or two before rinsing.

CHAMOMILE
(Anthemis nebilis)

Chamomile flowers, which are so pretty, are also excellent for our health. Chamomile grows wild, especially in meadows, creeping across the surface of the ground, rooting where they want, and dividing into branches and large, close-knit patches.

The leaves are finely divided, with the single daisy-like flower blossoming at the end of each branch. The scent of the herb is said to resemble that of an apple, and thus folklore gave it the name of "Earth Apple".

Double chamomile is found in many gardens, although from a medicinal point of view the wild flower is said to be a great value. Chamomile can be purchased in flower, tea bag, tincture, extract, or juice form.

It is an absolutely wonder herb for digestion. The flowers are prepared in a tea, one or two tablespoons to a cup of boiling water. Drink half a cupful at a time.

Chamomile also helps relieve stomach ache in babies and small children. Strain before adding it to a baby bottle, and always use it in a diluted form. Chamomile is an ancient remedy for children's diarrhea, and a wonderful aid to restful sleep.

It also makes an excellent insect repllent. Splash some chamomile tea on your exposed skin, face, arms and legs, before you go out and mosquitoes and other insects will leave you alone.

But be warned: Chamomile flowers grow on the ground and are sometimes accidentally picked along with ragweed. If you are allergic to ragweed, be very careful!

GINGER
(Zingiber offinale)

Ginger tea is an excellent aid in preventing colds, says Dr. Dian Dincin Buchman in her excellent book, *Herbal Medicine*, and recommends using a combination of peppermint, a pinch of ginger and a pinch of clove powder, or two bruised cloves. Ginger tea can be used to combat nausea and to stimulate the digestive organs. Ginger grows readily in the garden and is widely available in root form in Oriental groceries and fruit stores.

Grated ginger baths can help ease muscle and joint pain and improves sluggish circulation. Just drop a few granules of grated ginger in the bathtub. Don't use too much. Like cayenne, ginger quickly brings the blood to the surface.

To make ginger tea, use a pinch to a tablespoonful of the powder, or grate or slice the fresh root. Simmer in water until the brew turns yellowish. For pain, soak a cloth or a sponge in ginger tea and apply directly to the area of pain.

GINSENG
(Panax schinseng)

Ginseng is an excellent tonic and pick-me-up. Researchers say it sharpens memory, stops coughing, and helps prevent, and fight, colds. You can buy ginseng as a dried root, a tincture, a powder, or an extract.

To restore energy drop a pinch of ginseng powder in a cup of hot water and drink it. Or you can use a prepared ginseng tea extract, a capsule of powdered root, or chew on a piece of raw root.

Japanese scientists, principally Professor S. Shibata and Professor K. Takagi, claim that their experiments on mice proved that ginseng added to the diet increases — and speeds up — the ability to absorb information. And students at Uppsala University, in Sweden, who added ginseng to their daily diet, studied better, worked faster and scored consistently higher on tests than their peers.

Most of the peoples of the Far East areas of Asia consider ginseng root a medical miracle, a cure-all. They use it to treat a whole range of illnesses — from the common cold to arthritis, respiratory ailments like bronchitis and asthma, and inflammation of all kinds. Enthusiasts chew it as a root, add the powder to their tea, and use the extract in drinks and food.

BLACK MUSTARD
(Brassica nigra)

Considered one of the most important of all herbal medicines, black mustard is wonderful for preparing poultices to alleviate chest and other congestions. It is also an excellent ingredient in a hot footbath, to ease chest or nasal congestions and banish head-aches.

To make a mustard footbath, add about a tablespoonful of dried mustard powder to hot water. It will ease a cold in the head, a chest cough or a headache.

To make a mustard poultice, add one tablespoon of mustard to every four tablespoons of flour. The more flour, the weaker the plaster or poultice will be. Mix the ingredients in a bowl with a tiny amount of warm water, just enough to make a thick paste.

Fold two large, clean, white linen cloths (two large handker-chiefs will do), add the mustard paste and apply it to the con-gested chest or painful rheumatic area. If the patient has a deli-cate skin, apply a thin coating of olive or castor oil first.

BLADDERWRACK
(Fucus vesiculosus)

This is a seaweed which flourishes on coastlines all over the world. Anyone who has been to the seaside will recognize its branching fronds studded with little "bladders". When these are opened a thick jelly-like substance oozes out.

It is the presence of iodine in bladderwrack — it is also found in other seaweeds — which makes this herb particularly useful in treating scrofula, a tuberculosis of the lymphatic glands.

In the fishing villages of 19th century Yorkshire, England, many children suffered from dreadfully bowed legs, the result of an ail-ment called rickets, and being encouraged to walk at a very early age. Yet few of the adults had the deformity. The treatment was to combine a few drops of rum or gin with bladderwrack and rub it on the malformed legs until the condition eventually corrected itself.

British herbalist Mary Thorne Quelch, author of *Herbs for Daily Use*, wrote that the recipe required the gathering of a large quan-tity of the fresh seaweed, rinsing it four or five times to remove the salt water, then cutting it into inch long pieces.

"Put all into a bottle and add sufficient spirit and water in equal parts, to cover it," she wrote. "Either gin or rum may be used. Cork well and keep for a week, shaking the bottle each day. At the end of that time use as an embrocation. Do not strain. More of the spir-it and water may be added to the same herb." The same treat-ment is strongly recommended for rheumatism, joint and muscle pain, and lumbago.

The same preparation can also be used in any case of sprain. Quelch tells the story of a man who, when climbing sea-washed rocks on a remote coastline, slipped and sprained his leg so badly he thought it was broken. Lying helpless, he was in danger of drowning in the rising tide when he remembered the virtues of bladderwrack. Gathering the herb, he slit open the bladders with his knife, and rubbed his injured leg with their jelly-like contents. Within a few minutes, she recorded, he was able to hobble home.

Bladderwrack is also a safe means of slimming, wrote Quelch. "Being diuretic in its action, it removes superfluous moisture from the body by perfectly natural means. It is particularly recommended for those whose superabundant weight arises from rheumatic tendencies. The usual infusion should be prepared and taken in wineglassful size doses three times a day. Ask for seaweed pills at your local health store or herbalist."

PEPPERMINT AND SPEARMINT
(Mentha piperita and Mentha viridis)

Spearmint is that familiar mint found in many kitchens, and is distinguished from the peppermint by its smooth stems and the leaves being without foot-long stalks. Peppermint is familiar to us all, usually in the form of lozenges and cordials.

Try mint tea for headaches, and menstrual cramps. Use fresh or dried mint, from peppermint or spearmint, but the freshly gathered herb is most highly recommended.

Put a teaspoonful of dried mint or about a half dozen sprigs of freshly gathered herb, in a teacup. Fill with boiling water, and set a saucer on top for about five minutes to let the potion infuse properly. Then add a pinch of bicarbonate of soda, stir and sip while it is still very hot.

For cramps, add half a teaspoonful of ground ginger and the same amount of bicarbonate of soda to the mint before adding water. For nervous headaches, lie down in a darkened room and lay freshly gathered mint leaves on the forehead. Menthol, so often prescribed by herbalists in these cases, is obtained from peppermint although the fresh herb, as usual, is preferred by the experts.

Sufferers from asthma and ailments which cause breathing difficulties, wrote Mrs. Quelch, should use essence of mint, added to a half cup of warm water. This mixture should then be bottled and tightly corked. If there is shortness of breath, a few drops sprinkled on a piece of cloth and held to the mouth and nose, will bring speedy relief. The same mixture sprinkled on a pillow works well overnight. The pain of indigestion is quickly relieved by taking two to four drops of the oil of mint on a lump of sugar.

For rheumatic pains, swab the skin with oil of peppermint. It will provide relief instantly. A drop or two of the oil on a cotton ball will relieve toothache.

For small children suffering from diarrhea, a few sprigs of bruised peppermint should be laid on the pit of the abdomen. Or try half a teaspoonful of essence of peppermint in three tablespoons of warm water, wrote Mrs. Quelch.

RHUBARB
(Rheum rhaponticum)

Rhubarb is one of those strange plants that combine many different qualities. In small doses it acts as an astringent and will check a mild attack of diarrhea. In larger quantities it becomes a laxative. As a medicine it is best given in the form of powdered root, or an essence, and can be found in most health food stores.

The stem of the rhubarb makes a blood-purifying and wholesome food which, however, should be avoided by all prone to gout or any similiar ailment. The same rule holds true with rhubarb wine, an extremely soothing drink.

Note: The leaves of the rhubarb are toxic to some people.

The so-called *Turkey Rhubarb (Rheum palmatum)*, generally used in medicine, does not come from Turkey, despite the name. It works much the same as rhubarb, but is much stronger.

Rhubarb is used either as a powder or tincture, and though often used alone, it is frequently combined with other remedies. It is a very safe laxative, say herbalists, and can be found at your local supermarket produce counter or in pill form at most health stores.

COLTSFOOT
(Tussilago farfara)

Coltsfoot derives its name from the shape of its leaves, which resemble the hooves of a horse. The herb abounds on banks and ditch sides where the soil is predominantly gravelly or clay. On embankments and the sides of cliffs the plant binds the earth, but in gardens and fields it is regarded as a nuisance weed which is difficult to kill after it has properly taken root.

Writes Quelch: "The leaves are generally heart-shaped, but usually angular on the margins, with many irregular teeth. They do not appear until after the flowers are withered."

She adds: "The brillantly yellow flowers are placed singly upon thick, scaly stalks, and, opening in early spring, are amongst the earliest to decorate our banks and ditches. They are followed by the seeds, furnished with a long hairy pappus which enables the wind to carry them away and so distribute them over the country."

Coltsfoot cannot be praised too highly as a medicine for the relief of coughs, or any irritation of the lungs and air passages. The usual infusion of the leaves, according to Quelch, should be prepared and taken in teacuful doses whenever the cough is troublesome. It may be sweetened to taste, preferably with honey.

Another excellent recipe for the soothing of any cough, Quelch advises, is prepared by simmering an ounce of licorice root in three pints of water till reduced to a pint, and pouring into a jug in which an ounce of coltsfoot and a sliced lemon have been placed. Stir well, sweeten with honey, allow to get cold, then strain. Drink freely as required.

"Many bronchitis or asthma sufferers have benefited from smoking what is known as herbal tobacco, and of this coltsfoot is the chief ingredient," Quelch writes.

She adds: "Herbal tobacco may be brought from any good herbalist, but many smokers prefer to prepare their own, omitting some of the usual herbs or increasing the proportion of others as their individual tastes may dictate. The usual ingredients are buckbean, betony, eyebright, rosemary, thyme, lavender and chamomile flowers."

Of these, equal parts can be used, Quelch explains, or the proportions altered to suit the taste of the smoker. The dried herbs should be rubbed between the hands until they are reduced to a fine powder and thoroughly mixed. Take as much coltsfoot as needed to equal the quality of all the others combined, reduce to a fine powder and mich with the other herbs. For proper storage, place the powder in a sealed tin, either as pipe tobacco or as cigarettes.

Ode to Garlic

Sudden, it comes for you
in the cave of yourself where you know
and are lifted by important events.
Say you are dining and it happens:
soaring like an eagle, you are
pierced by the message from the midst of life.
Memory—what holds the days together—
touches
your tongue. It is from deep in the earth
and it reaches out kindly, saying, "Hello,
Old Friend."
It makes us all alike, all offspring of powerful
forces, part of one great embrace of
democracy,
united across every boundary.
You walk out generously, giving it back
in a graceful wave, what you've been
given.
Like a child again, you breathe on the
world, and it shines.

William Stafford
Poet Laureate of the State of Oregon

10 Great Garlic Recipes

The most wondrous substances nature has to offer you come in the form of wholesome food. They don't need any magical healing properties beyond the nourishment and sustenance they supply — fiber, vitamins, minerals and other elements. They are the stuff of life and there's little else you require for health, happiness, and a long and productive time on earth.

Plant foods are the best friends you have and Mother Nature intended you to eat them in copious quantities every day. If you're eating it, and it came out of the ground as a root, stalk, stem or leaf, it is almost certainly high in fiber, free of dangerous, artery-clogging fats and cholesterol, extremely low in calories and loaded with goodness — the same goes for whole grain foods such as rice, oats, corn, rye, millet, etc.

Health agencies, researchers, the National Academy of Sciences — your family doctor — all recommend a diet that is high in fiber. A diet in which the calories are derived from 60 percent carbohydrates, 10 percent protein and no more than 30 percent fat, can protect you from serious illnesses such as cancer, heart disease and diabetes. Other experts recommend even less fat — as little as 20 or in some cases 10 percent of total caloris from fat. fat.

You may wonder what all that means.

You can place yourself in the ballpark and not have to worry or count or calculate precisely if you follow a few, simple steps. First, eat cereal with some oat bran sprinkled on it for breakfast, with a piece of fruit and some toast or a roll. Eat two salads a day, one at lunch and the other at dinner. Consume at least three cups of raw vegetables a day; plan one meatless meal every week; and limit the amount of meat you eat to four ounces a day.

This will enable you to eat more than ever before, and weigh less! This is the way that nature, and your body, intended you to eat. This is the natural way.

Bearing that in mind, here are some wondrous recipes. L. John Harris, author of *The Book of Garlic*, says, "There are a number of recipes that treat garlic as it should be treated — as a vegetable and not merely a spice, herb, seasoning or flavoring." He suggests a number of creative ways to bake, boil, sautee and broil garlic. The results are delicious and cooking mellows the bulb. Herewith some excellent recipes from his *The Book of Garlic*:

Roasted Garlic

10—12 large garlic cloves, peeled
2 tbs butter
1 tbs peanut oil
1 tbs olive oil
Salt to taste
Pinch of white pepper

Heat the butter, peanut and olive oils in a casserole over medium heat. Put in peeled cloves, side by side, and make sure they are well coated. Bake at 350 degrees for 20 minutes, basting from time to time. Add salt and pepper. Serve as an appetizer with toast or as a vegetable side dish.

Charcoal Roasted Whole Garlic

Middle Eastern Specialty. Place whole bulbs of garlic directly, basted with oil, salt and pepper, in white hot but not flaming coals. When they're lightly browned, they're ready. Allow the bulbs to cool and break off the cloves. A taste bud tingler!

Halved Heads of Garlic in Sauce

A delicious side dish with chicken.
4 heads of garlic
1 tbs olive oil
2 tbs butter
1 cup chicken stock
1 cup white wine
Pinch of thyme
Salt and pepper

Cut the four heads of garlic in half. Heat the oil and butter in a saucepan and saute the bulbs cut side down in moderate heat until the garlic meat begins to brown. Now add the chicken stock, wine and herbs. Cover the pan with a tight lid and braise over low heat until liquid is reduced and thickened and the garlic cloves are soft when poked with a knife. Serve the halved heads cut side up on the plate and spoon some of the stock over each. Use the sauce over chicken pieces also. Eat the garlic like an artichoke, using your teeth and lips to pull the puree out of the skins.

Garlic Puree

2 dozen garlic cloves or more
1 tbs olive oil
Pinch of salt and pepper
Pinch of the herbs of your choice

Place whole, unpeeled cloves in a pot of boiling water for about 20 minutes or until clove meat is very soft. Drain and cool. When cool, remove skins and place cloves in a food processor or blender. Puree, adding salt, pepper, herbs and olive oil. Fill a glass jar and refrigerate. Use to thicken and flavor sauces, soups, stews, dressings and dips. Spread on croutons and serve with soups and salads. It can also be a sandwich spread for leftover meats.

Fancy Pesto Genovese

1 cup fresh basil leaves, washed and dry
4 spinach leaves
6 sprigs of parsley
3 sprigs of marjoram
½ cup pine nuts
4 cloves garlic
¾ cup Parmesan cheese OR
⅓ cup Parmesan with ⅓ cup Romano cheese
½ cup olive oil
¼ tsp salt

Mix in an electric blender, adding the oil a little bit at a time. Serve over hot, fresh pasta.

Parsley Salad with Garlic Dressing

3 large bunches parsley
¼ cup salad oil
Juice of 1 large lemon
5 cloves fresh garlic, crushed
1 tsp salt
½ tsp pepper
1 lb mushrooms, sliced
4 tbs grated Parmesan

Rinse parsley thoroughly, remove stems and separate into small clusters. Combine oil, lemon juice, garlic, salt and pepper. Mix. Toss parsley and Parmesan. Add mushrooms and refrigerate until ready to serve. The parsley neutralizes garlic breath.

By: Soledad Zuzuarregui, Tucson, AZ

Technicolor Garlique Shrimp

1 full head garlic (approx 12 cloves)
16 large shrimp
3 large bell peppers (red, green and yellow)
3 tbs vegetable oil
¼ lb butter
¼ cup Chinese chili paste
2 cups cooked rice

Blanch garlic cloves in boiling water three minutes. Drain, peel and slice. Set aside. Peel and devein shrimp and slice in half lengthwise. Set aside. Cut peppers into ½-inch strips. Heat oil and butter in large heavy skillet, saute peppers, tossing and stirring for one minute. Add shrimp and continue to toss and stir until shrimp turns pink. Stir in sliced garlic and chili paste. Serve over hot rice.

By: Lori Shula, Reseda, CA

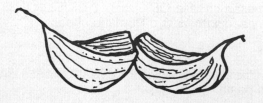

Healthy, Hot and Garlicky Wings

2 lbs chicken wings (approximately 15 wings)
3 heads fresh garlic
1 cup olive oil plus 1 tablespoon
10-15 drops Tabasco
1 cup grated Parmesan cheese
1 cup Italian style breadcrumbs
1 tsp black pepper

Preheat oven to 375°. Disjoint chicken wings, discarding tips, rinse and pat dry. Separate garlic cloves and peel. Place garlic, olive oil and tabasco in blender or food processor and puree. Combine Parmesan, breadcrumbs and pepper in a plastic bag. Dip wings in the garlic puree and roll in breadcrumb mixture, one at a time, coating thoroughly. Coat a shallow non-stick baking pan with oil and add wings in a single layer. Drizzle with remaining garlic puree and sprinkle with any remaining breadcrumb mixture. Bake for 45 to 60 minutes until brown and crisp.

By: Winifred Harano, Los Angeles, CA

Betty Jayne's Garlic Soup

4 tbs olive oil
30 large fresh garlic cloves, chopped
2 cans chicken broth, about 1 qt
2 cups water
1 tsp each salt and water
2 bay leaves
1 fresh Jalapeno pepper, seeded and chopped
1 cup whipping cream
12 slices French bread
Parmesan cheese grated

In saucepan, heat oil on medium. Add garlic and saute until soft and golden. Add chicken broth, water, salt, pepper, bay leaves, and Jalapeno pepper. Simmer 5 minutes. Pour into blender and puree. Return to saucepan. Stir in cream and heat through. Toast bread lightly. Sprinkle with Parmesan cheese and broil 3 minutes or until cheese is golden and bubbly. Serve toast in soup.

By: Betty Jane Jones, Longview, MA

John Bautista-Style
Garlicky Stuffed Chicken Wings

12 chicken wings (approximately two pounds)
½ lb Chinese-type barbequed pork (or cooked ham)
1 medium sized garlic bulb
1 qt cooking oil
Tempura batter

Remove large bone in chicken wing, being careful not to cut the outer skin. Stuff cavity with meat and garlic (garlic to taste). Dip stuffed wings in tempura batter. Fry in very hot oil. Cook until golden brown. Remove from oil and drain on paper towels. Serve hot. Very good when served with dipping sauce.

By: John Bautista

Thirty-Clove Chicken

2 broiler-fryer chickens, cut-up
4 tbs olive oil
2 tbs butter
1 tbs flour
1 can chicken broth
30 cloves fresh garlic, peeled
1 cup rice
Fresh chives
Fresh parsley minced

Brown chicken in 2 tablespoons oil and butter. Remove from pan and stir in flour, then broth and garlic. Bring to a boil, return chicken to pan and simmer, covered for 45 minutes. Saute rice in remaining 2 tablespoons of oil until rice is opaque. Add to chicken, easing into liquid with fork. Cover and simmer for another 25 minutes. Just prior to serving, stir in herbs. Serves 8.

By: Leah Jackson, Marshfield, MA

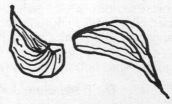

Broiled Garlic and Lemon Chicken

6 oz lemon juice (from 3 lemons)
¼ cup melted butter (or half butter & half corn oil)
3 large cloves garlic, crushed or minced
½ tsp oregano
Salt and pepper (to taste)
2 tsp corn oil
1—3 lb broiler-fryer chicken cut into quarters

Mix the lemon juice, butter, garlic, oregano, salt and pepper. Pre-heat the broiler and brush pan with 2 teaspoons of oil. Broil chicken, skin side down, for 25 minutes until golden brown, basting with garlic butter sauce. Keep chicken about 12 inches from the source of heat. Turn chicken pieces, skin side up; broil 20 minutes longer, basting frequently, until chicken is fork tender. Garnish with lemon slices and parsley if desired.

By: Karen Christopher, Gilroy, CA

Gilroy Chili

3 cloves fresh garlic, minced
2 large onions, finely chopped
2 tbs olive oil
2 lbs ground beef
1 can (4 oz.) green chiles
1 cup canned stewed tomatoes
2 cups beef stock
1 tbs chili powder
1 tbs ground cumin
1 tsp salt
¼ tsp pepper

In a large skillet, slowly brown the garlic and onions in olive oil; stir and cook until tender. Raise heat, add meat and cook until done. Add all other ingredients. Cover and reduce heat. Cook about 45 minutes more. Remove grease or add a small amount of cornstarch to absorb it.

By: David B. Swope, Redondo Beach, CA

Eggplant Antipasta

4-6 eggplants (Chinese or Japanese)
4 tomatoes, chopped
1 bulb garlic, crushed or finely chopped
Fresh basil, finely chopped or dried
Olive oil
Salt and Pepper to taste
Parmesan cheese, grated (optional)

Cut eggplant in half, lengthwise, then again crosswise so you end up with 4 pieces. Make a couple of slits on the meat of the eggplant without cutting through to the skin. Stuff chopped tomatoes into the slits of the eggplant, place garlic on top and sprinkle with basil. Sprinkle with Parmesan cheese, if so desired. Drizzle with lots of olive oil. Bake in a pan at 350° F. for 25-30 minutes.

By: Rudy and Gloria Melone

Veal Garlic Chop

1 veal chop (approx. 14 oz)
1 tbs crushed, peeled black peppercorns
Salt to taste
2 tbs butter
1 tbs olive oil
1 green pepper
1 red bell pepper
1 medium onion
6 cloves fresh garlic, minced
1 tsp finely chopped fresh parsley

Rub the black peppercorns into the entire surface of the veal chop and add salt. In a heavy skillet, combine the butter and oil, heat on high; add the veal and reduce heat to medium. Cook for about 7 minutes, then turn and brown the other side. Meanwhile, remove the seeds and membranes from the peppers. Slice peppers and onion into julienne strips and add to skillet with veal. Add a pinch of salt.

Spread garlic evenly over chop; cover skillet and cook about 10 minutes, stirring vegetables occasionally, until tender. To serve, arrange peppers and onion on plate, top with veal chop and sprinkle with parsley.

Serves one. Double everything for two, triple for three, quadruple for four and so on.

By: David Lindley, Union City, GA

Garlic Plumped Chicken

3 heads fresh garlic
1 chicken (3½ to 4 lbs)
¾ lbs fresh mushrooms
8 tbs unsalted butter
Salt and pepper
¼ cup chicken stock
¼ cup marsala (or port or red wine)
¼ cup heavy cream
Juices from cavity of roasted chicken

Wrap garlic in foil and roast in preheated 400° oven about 30 minutes or until garlic is cooked and soft. Cool, then squeeze out pulp of cloves and set aside. Rinse chicken and pat dry. With breast side up, beginning at the neck end, separate the skin from flesh, loosening as far into the legs and wings as possible without tearing skin. This creates a pocket for the stuffing. Set chicken aside. Clean mushrooms and finely chop (a food processor works best).

Saute in 2 tablespoons butter over high heat until all moisture has evaporated, stirring and taking care not to burn. Cool. Combine ⅔ garlic pulp, mushrooms, and remaining 6 tablespoons butter. Mix thoroughly; add salt and pepper to taste. To stuff chicken, fill a pastry bag (use a medium tip) with garlic mixture. Insert point under skin and pump filling into pocket, spreading evenly with fingers.

Rub outside of chicken with a little butter and sprinkle with fresh ground pepper. Place chicken breast side up in a roasting pan with a rack and roast at 400° for approximately 1½ hours until juices in thigh run clear. Reserve juices from cavity; carefully cut up chicken into serving pieces, and keep warm.

Prepare sauce by combining remaining third of garlic pulp and reserved juices with stock, wine and cream in a small saucepan over high heat. Stir until thickened. Serve with chicken.

Makes 4 servings

By: Joseph Bonello, San Francisco, CA

Garlic Onion Bake

3 oz soda crackers, about 35 crackers, rolled fine
3 oz Ritz crackers, about 35 crackers, rolled fine
10 tbs (1 ¼ sticks) unsalted butter, melted
3 large red onions
1 cup chopped fresh garlic
8 oz sharp white cheddar cheese (no dyes)
2 eggs
1 ½ cups milk

Place crackers in a bowl and pour all but two tablespoons butter over. Mix well. Press half the cracker mixture on bottom of 9 x 11 inch baking dish.

Slice onions thin and saute with garlic in remaining butter until translucent but not brown. Place in baking dish and spread over crackers. Grate cheese and sprinkle over garlic onion mixture. Beat eggs. Pour this mixture over cheese and sprinkle remaining crackers on top. Bake at 350 degrees F. for 30 minutes.

By: Ira J. Jacobson, Oakland, CA

Poached Garlic With Butter

Place peeled or unpeeled cloves in gently boiling water. Let them simmer until soft, testing one with a fork. Strain off water and put butter (about a tablespoon per five cloves) and garlic into a warm pan. Simply serve with the melted butter or saute until lightly browned. Add salt and pepper to taste and serve on toast or French bread as a side dish with meat, fish or fowl.

By: John Lloyd

Linguine With Caramelized Garlic

3 heads fresh garlic
3 tbs olive oil
1 tbs chopped fresh thyme
⅓ cup chicken stock (if using canned, use regular, not double strength)
Salt and pepper to taste
6 oz linguine
2 eggs, beaten
3 oz freshly grated Parmesan cheese

Separate garlic cloves. Immerse in boiling water for 30 seconds and peel. Heat oil in large saute pan over medium-low heat. Add garlic. Reduce heat to low and very slowly saute garlic until golden brown. Stir frequently. Be careful not to burn garlic. It will take approximately 20 minutes for the garlic to reach this state. Stir in fresh thyme. Cook 2 minutes longer. Add chicken stock, salt and pepper. Simmer 5 minutes.

Meanwhile, cook linguine according to package directions. Drain. Toss linguine with eggs. Add to saute pan and toss with Parmesan cheese. Adjust seasonings. Serve immediately.

Makes 3-4 servings

By: Kimra Foster, San Jose, CA

Ambrosial Grape Leaves

1 jar grape leaves
1 onion, chopped
2 tbs butter or olive oil
1 ½ lbs ground lamb
1-2 heads fresh garlic, peeled and chopped
Salt and pepper
4-10 oz pine nuts (pignolas)
2 cups seedless raisins
2-3 tbs sugar
6 tbs cinnamon
1 stick (8 oz) butter, melted

Rinse grape leaves, cut off stems and lay flat on work surface. Saute onion in butter or olive oil until translucent. Add lamb, crumbling as you cook, until done. Stir in garlic, and season with salt and pepper to taste. Remove from heat and add pine nuts, raisins, sugar and cinnamon. Place 2 to 3 tablespoonsful of the mixture in the center of each grape leaf. Fold each leaf over filling and roll up like a cigar. Preheat oven to 350°. Fill a baking dish with the stuffed grape leaves in a single layer and dribble melted butter over them. Bake for 20 minutes and serve hot.

Makes 10 servings

By: Elaine Corrington, Los Angeles, CA

Homemade Italian Sausage

9 lbs Boston butt pork roast, boned
3 oz salt
3 tbs black pepper
¼ cup fresh garlic, finely chopped
3 tbs crushed red chili pepper
Casings — pork small intestines
Optional:
2 tbs fennel
1 tbs oregano

Grind pork roast with a coarse grind sausage blade. Add salt, black pepper, garlic, chili peppers and the options desired. Knead this mixture thoroughly for at least 10 minutes. When mixed properly, the mixture will stick to your hand for 3 or 4 seconds when held upside down.

Wash the casings thoroughly in water, inside and out. Tie one end closed and then pack the ingredients inside the casing tightly, making sure to remove all air and filling the voids. Tie the other end closed.

About every 4 or 5 inches, pinch the filled casing together and double the end back through in a looping motion. This will divide your sausage into individual connected pieces.

With a fork, prick each segment 3 or 4 times. Place the sausage in an uncovered container and refrigerate them for 3 days. This allows the ingredients to "marry". Sausage can also be dried or frozen.

By: Bob McHam, Don Gage and Dick Bozzo

Two Guys from Calabria
Rainy Sunday Super Stuffed Shells

2 tbs olive oil
3 cloves garlic
¾ lb ground veal
¾ lb ground pork
1 10 oz package frozen chopped spinach
1 cup parsley, finely chopped
1 cup bread crumbs
2 eggs, beaten

3 cloves minced garlic
3 tbs Parmesan cheese, grated
Salt to taste
1 12 oz package jumbo pasta shells
3 cups of your favorite tomato sauce

Mix ground veal and ground pork together. In a large skillet, heat the olive oil over medium heat and saute three whole cloves of garlic until brown. Remove and discard garlic, add the veal and pork mixture and lightly brown. Drain excess fat and set aside to cool.

In a large mixing bowl, combine the cooked chopped spinach, parsley, bread crumbs, eggs, minced garlic and cheese. Blend well and salt to taste. Add cooled browned meat and mix thoroughly.

Bring 3 quarts of salted water to a full boil. Carefully add the jumbo pasta shells. Cook the shells for 5 to 7 minutes. The shells should be undercooked for ease of handling. Drain and immediately rinse under plenty of cold water.

Preheat oven to 375° F. Generously coat the bottom of an 8" x 11" baking dish with some of the tomato sauce. Using a teaspoon, fill the cooked shells with the stuffing and arrange decoratively in the baking dish. Spoon additional tomato sauce over each stuffed shell and cover the baking dish with aluminum foil. Bake for 35 to 45 minutes.

Serves 9 to 12

By: Paul and Ernie Filice

Pasta with Garlic, Butter and Cheese

A simple and delicious way to serve a nutritious meal quickly. Melt the butter in a sauce pan and add 4 to 6 cloves of garlic which you've mashed until they're transparent. Simmer 2 to 3 minutes but don't let the butter brown. Pour over hot pasta and grate fresh Parmesan cheese on top.

Nancy's Glorious Garlic Tart

Pastry crust (recipe follows)
3 heads fresh garlic, cloves separated and peeled
2 tsp Dijon-style mustard
1 cup grated Gruyere cheese
1 egg
¼ cup heavy cream
1 tsp nutmeg
¼ tsp pepper

Half fill a large saucepan with water. Add garlic cloves and bring to a boil. Drain garlic, and repeat process with fresh water. Drain and reserve garlic. With back of spoon, smear mustard across bottom of pastry crust, which can be hot from oven or at room temperature. Distribute cheese evenly inside crust. In a food processor, puree reserved garlic with egg, cream, nutmeg and pepper for 30 seconds. Pour garlic mixture over cheese. Bake tart at 350° for 25 minutes, until filling is firm. Serve hot or at room temperature.

Makes 8 servings

Pastry Crust

1 ½ cups all purpose flour
1 tsp sugar
1 tsp salt
1 stick (8 oz.) frozen butter, cut into 6 pieces
¼ cup ice water

Preheat oven to 350°. In food processor, combine flour, sugar, salt and butter until mixture looks crumbly. With motor running, slowly add water. Mixture will gather in a ball. Wrap dough in plastic wrap and refrigerate for at least half an hour. Butter and flour inside of a 9-inch tart pan which has a removable bottom. Roll out dough to fit into pan. Trim edges. Line dough with foil and fill center with pie weights or dried beans. Bake for 20 minutes. Remove foil and weights. Continue baking crust for additional 10 minutes, until crust begins to brown.

By: Nancy Ash, San Francisco, CA

Spaghettaccini Carolini

1 lb spaghetti noodles
4 tbs oil
¼ lb. butter
24 cloves fresh garlic, peeled and chopped
1 lb fresh jumbo shrimp, peeled and butterflied
1 red bell pepper, thinly sliced
1 bunch broccoli, cut into serving size spears
2 cups fresh mushrooms
1 cup chopped fresh parsley
1 cup chopped green onions
1 tbs dried red pepper
2 tbs flour
½ cup dry white wine
1 pint heavy cream
1 small wedge (about 3 oz) Parmesan cheese, grated
Salt to taste

Cook noodles according to package directions in boiling water with 2 tablespoons oil. Meanwhile, melt butter in large skillet over medium high heat. Add chopped garlic and shrimp; cook until shrimp turns pink, but do not allow garlic to brown. Set aside. In another skillet, over medium high heat, stir fry red bell pepper and broccoli in remaining 2 tablespoons oil. Cook until crisp-tender. Drain and set aside. Add mushrooms, half the parsley, onions and red pepper to garlic and shrimp; saute for one minute. Add flour, mix thoroughly and add wine.

Simmer for about 30 seconds, then add cream and heat thoroughly, stirring. Drain noodles and add to sauce with half the grated cheese. Toss gently until noodles are well coated and cheese is melted. Salt lightly. If sauce is too thin, continue heating until sauce reduces to a creamy consistency. If sauce is too thick, add cream. Gently toss in the stir-fried vegetables. Garnish with remaining chopped parsley and grated cheese and serve immediately.

Serves 6

By: Robert J. Dyer

Patrician Escargots

4 heads fresh garlic
½ cup olive oil
½ cup butter
1 onion finely chopped
1 tsp finely chopped fresh or dried rosemary
¼ tsp ground thyme
2 dashes nutmeg
Salt and pepper to taste
24 large canned snails
½ cup chopped parsley
24 medium to large fresh mushrooms
12 pieces thin sliced white bread

Peel garlic and chop into fine pieces. Place olive oil and butter in a frying pan over medium heat. When butter is melted, add onion, garlic, rosemary and thyme. Then add nutmeg, salt and pepper. Reduce heat to low, and add snails and parsley; simmer for 30 minutes. While snails are simmering, clean and remove stems from mushrooms. Arrange mushroom caps upside down in a 2-inch deep baking dish and place one snail into each mushroom cap. Pour garlic mixture over snails, cover with foil and bake at 350° for 30 minutes. While snails are baking, cut the crust off bread slices and cut each slice into 4 squares. Toast bread. Serve with Escargots.

Makes 4 servings

By: Pat Trainchero, Gilroy, CA

Scampi Alla "Fireman Chef"

1 lb large prawns
8 sprigs fresh parsley
⅓ cup clarified butter
4 tbs minced garlic
6 scallions, thinly sliced
Juice of a lemon (approximately 2 tbs)
¼ cup dry white wine
Salt and freshly ground pepper, to taste
Lemon slices for garnish

Shell and devein the prawns. Rinse and set aside. Reserve a few nice sprigs of parsley for garnish and mince the rest. Heat the clarified butter in a large saute pan over medium heat. Lightly saute the garlic for 1 to 2 minutes, being careful not to let it brown. Add the prawns, scallions, lemon juice and wine. Cook the mixture until the prawns turn pink and firm, a minute or two on each side. Be careful not to overcook.

At the last minute, add the minced parsely and season with salt and pepper. Serve the scampi on individual shells or small gratin dishes, garnished with a slice or two of lemon and a fresh parsley sprig.

By: Jim Neil

Garlic Chicken Pineapple
1 head fresh garlic, peeled
1 piece (1 inch square) fresh ginger, peeled
5 tbs vegetable oil
9 black peppercorns
5 cardomon pods
5 whole cloves
1 stick cinnamon
1 large onion (preferably red), chopped
1 chicken, skinned and cut up
2 potatoes, peeled and diced (optional)
1 can sliced pineapple, drained and cut in triangular pieces

In blender, grind garlic and ginger to form a smooth paste; add a little water for good consistency, but not too much. Heat oil and add peppercorns, cardomon, cloves and cinnamon, cooking until light golden in color. Add garlic-ginger paste and cook about 5 minutes, stirring constantly. If this "masala" is sticking to the pan, reduce heat to medium. Once chicken is browned, add about 1 cup water and deglaze pan. Reduce heat to medium low, cover pan and let chicken cook 50 minutes or until tender. Add potatoes, if desired, after chicken has cooked 20 minutes. Just before serving, add pineapple.

Makes 4 servings

By: B.K. Kermani, San Jose, CA

Gloria's Lamb Stew

This is lamb stew with a difference — chili peppers, garlic and fresh cilantro are the seasonings.

1 cup fresh cilantro leaves (coriander)
1 whole head fresh garlic, peeled
2 or 3 fresh hot red or green peppers, seeded
½ cup olive oil
2 medium onions, finely chopped
4 lb lean boneless lamb, cut into 1-inch cubes
Salt and freshly ground pepper to taste
⅔ cup fresh orange juice
⅓ cup lime or lemon juice water
2 lb potatoes, peeled and sliced
1 lb fresh green peas, shelled or 2 pkg (10 oz each) frozen

In blender or food processor puree cilantro, garlic and peppers; set aside. Heat oil in casserole or Dutch oven and saute onions until soft. Stir in cilantro mixture and cook for a minute or two longer. Add lamb pieces and cook for about 5 minutes, turning to coat with sauce. Season to taste with salt and a generous amount of pepper. Add orange and lime or lemon juice and enough water to cover, about 1 ½ cups. Cover and simmer until lamb is tender, about 1 ½ hours. If desired, this dish may be refrigerated at this point in order to solidify and remove any excess fat. Let stand to bring to room temperature before heating. Boil potatoes and peas separately in salted water until tender. Drain and add to casserole. Bring casserole to a simmer and cook just long enough to heat through.

Makes 4 to 5 servings.

By: Gloria Park, Los Gatos, CA

Desserts made with garlic? Well, why not? Everyone who tasted them agreed they were delicious and would even be better with more garlic!

Garlic Chip Cookies

10 cloves fresh garlic
Boiling water
½ cup maple syrup
1 cup butter, softened
¾ cup brown sugar
¾ cup sugar
2 eggs
1 tsp vanilla
½ tsp salt
2 ¼ cups chocolate chips
½ cup chopped nuts
2 ½ cups flour
1 tsp baking soda

Drop garlic cloves into boiling water for about 5 minutes until tender. Peel and chop garlic and soak in maple syrup for 20 minutes. Meanwhile, cream butter, sugars, eggs and vanilla together until light and fluffy. Combine flour, baking soda and salt. Add to cream mixture. Then stir in chocolate chips and nuts. Drain garlic, and add to cookie batter. Blend well. Drop cookie batter by tablespoons onto ungreased cookie sheet about 2 inches apart. Bake at 375° for 8 to 10 minutes, until lightly browned. Remove from oven and cool on racks.

Makes 5 dozen cookies

By: Michele Sciortino, San Diego, CA

During the First Garlic Festival, *Digger Dan's,* a Gilroy restaurant, featured this unusual dessert on their menu. Although the recipe calls for quite a lot of garlic, it is a light and flavorful dessert.

Garlic Pudding

2 heads fresh garlic
1 ½ cups cold water
1 cup sugar
1 envelope unflavored gelatin
¼ cup lemon juice
1 tsp lemon peel, grated
2 egg whites
¼ tsp nutmeg
Custard sauce (recipe below)
¼ tsp salt
¼ cup lemon juice

Wrap garlic heads in foil and bake until done (soft). Remove from foil and boil in water until flavor is transferred from bulbs to water and water is reduced to about 1¼ cups garlic water. In saucepan combine sugar, gelatin and salt. Add ½ cup garlic water; stir until dissolved and remove from heat. Add remaining ¾ cup garlic water, lemon juice and lemon peel. Chill until partially set. Turn into large bowl. Add egg whites and beat with electric mixer until mixture begins to hold its shape. Turn into mold. Chill until firm. Unmold and garnish with sprinkles of nutmeg and custard sauce.

Custard Sauce

4 egg yolks, beaten
¼ cup sugar
2 cups milk
Dash salt

In heavy saucepan, mix egg yolks with sugar, milk and salt. Cook over low heat until mixture coats spoon. Cool and serve.

By: Judith M. Bozzo, Gilroy, CA

11 Postscript for Good Health

What you eat and the way you eat it can make all the difference to your health — and as we have already stressed, it can truly make the difference between life and death.

Remember that proteins, fats, carbohydrates, vitamins, minerals and fiber are the essential foundation of a sound, well balanced diet.

Whole foods differ in their nutrient content, and that is why consuming a wide variety of foods is essential to provide you with a proper nutritional balance.

In simple terms, here is precisely what each of these building blocks gives you:

● Carbohydrates are fuels. Grains, fruits, peas and beans, nuts and vegetables are rich in natural starches and sugars. These are the best, cleanest, and most efficient sources of energy for your body.

● Fiber acts as a transport mechanism, keeping bulk moving from one end of the digestive system to the other, cleaning the intestines, gathering waste and eliminating it quickly and efficiently.

● Fats insulate you, build cells and make your metabolism function. There are three types: *saturated fats* (mainly from meats, dairy and packaged foods, processed or convenience foods) which contribute to heart disease; *polyunsaturated fats* and *monounsaturated fats.* These last two are obtained from vegetable sources.

● Proteins build and repair cells, and maximize your metabolism, which regulates the body's efficiency. Even though most of us believe the only source of protein is meats, eggs and cheeses, it's important to note that all vegetables and fruits have some protein, without that life threatening saturated fat.

● Minerals build bones and keep them strong, regulate body fluid levels and composition and release energy.

● Vitamins keep your body chemistry in balance. All but two of essential vitamins come from your food — the action of sunlight on your skin produces vitamin D and micro-organisms in the bowel produce vitamin K.

● Stick with whole, fresh or lightly processed foods and choose twice as many plant foods (such as fruits, vegetables and grains) as animal foods (meats, eggs and cheeses).

Eight Steps to Health

Sometimes good dietary advice can sound complicated. So let's map out a set of quite straightforwad and simple guidelines for healthy eating together. In this way we will increase the opportunities to let the wonders of garlic and vinegar do the most good.

1. Eat plenty of fiber. Switch from eggs to cereal for breakfast. Add toast, or a bagel or muffin or roll. Snack on these breads midmorning and mid-afternoon. Choose dark breads over white. Breads won't make you fat — fat will — because they are filling and satisfying, and low in calories. Whole grains, pastas, rice and cornmeal are wonderfully loaded down with fiber, as are all the wonderful fruits and vegetables.

2. Promise yourself to use these liberally. Eat at least four servings of vegetables (two of these servings should be raw, if at all possible) two fruits, and at least one serving of leafy green vegetables (such as spinach or dark green lettuce) every day. Recent data from the National Cancer Institute indicate that people who do eat vegetables are far less likely to develop colon cancer — which accounts for so many, many deaths every year all over the world.

3. And if you follow the advice in Step 2 above you will leave far less room for harmful rich, fatty foods. And that is so important for you, because cutting down on fats is the third point of your plan.

Try substituting peas and beans, served over rice or toast, instead of meat at least two meals a week. Prepare two or three fish meals and one completely vegetarian meal every week. Try vegetables, grains or a combination of the two. Choose chicken, turkey and other poultry over red meat and cheese. Whatever you do avoid fast-food restaurants and those all too convenient packaged snacks.

4. Slash your sugar intake. Sorry, but this step is absolutely essential. Use sugar, sparingly, as a flavoring rather than as a food. Just say *NO* to cookies, cakes and pies. Try to choose the new fruit spreads sweetened with natural fruit juices, over sugar loaded jellies, jams and preserves. Try substituting fruit juices or sparkling water instead of sweetened soft drinks, and leave the sugar out of coffee and tea.

5. Stop using salt. Don't add any when you are cooking, and simply remove the salt shaker from the table. That way all temptation is out of sight. Quite simply, nearly all of us get far too much sodium. Try using herbs and spices, fresh ginger, horseradish, lemon juice, vinegar, yeast extract and other flavorings to season foods instead.

6. Cut back on the consumption of processed foods. If it comes in a cellophane or tin foil bag, a box or a styrofoam container, it's unlikely to be high in nutrition. It might taste good, but it is likely to make you fat, clog your arteries, make you feel under-par and it may also give you pimples.

7. If you use alcohol, limit your intake to two drinks a day.

8. If you are overweight, shed enough to reach your ideal weight level. Ask a dietician for help.

Now that you have all of the background on the eating habits that are absolutely vital for your best health, you'll know how to get the most out of these astonishing twins, garlic and vinegar, and these other dazzling wonders of nature that we have just introduced you to.

And remember that there are more of these natural wonders out there. Consult some of the books we recommend in our reading list at the end of this book. You will find in these, far more detail about the remarkable world of natural foods and natural living than we can possibly cover here.

But we earnestly hope that what we have been able to share with you here will help you enjoy, enthusiastically and in good health, this marvellous gift of life.

Recommended
Reading

Buchman, Dian Dincin, PhD; *Herbal Medicine: The Natural Way to Get Well; (David McKay Company, Inc., New York: 1979),* $10.95.

Carper, Jean; The Food Pharmacy, (Bantam, New York: 1988), $18.95.

Carroll, David; *The Complete Book of Natural Medicines,* (Summit Books, New York: 1980), $17.95.

The Gilroy Garlic Festival Association, Inc.; *The Complete Garlic Lovers' Cook Book,* (Celestial Arts, Berkeley, California: 1987), $19.95.

Harris, Lloyd John; *The Book of Garlic,* (Aris Books/Addison Wesley, Reading, Massachusetts: 1974, 1978, 1979), $11.95 and *The Official Garlic Lovers Handbook,* (Aris Books, Berkeley, California: 1986), $7.95.

Jarvis, DeForest, Clinton, MD; *Folk Medicine*; (Henry Holt and Company, New York: 1958).

Mindell, Earl, PhD; *Vitamin Bible*; (Warner, New York: 1979), $3.95.

Olshevsky, Moshe, CA, PhD; Noy, Shlomo, MD; Zwang, Moses, PhD; *The Manual of Natural Therapy*; (Facts on File, New York: 1989), $24.95.

Stanway, Dr. Penny; *Foods for Common Ailments;* (Fireside, New York: 1989), $10.95.